T0264342

Angioedema

Editor

MARC A. RIEDL

IMMUNOLOGY AND ALLERGY CLINICS OF NORTH AMERICA

www.immunology.theclinics.com

Consulting Editor
STEPHEN A. TILLES

August 2017 • Volume 37 • Number 3

ELSEVIER

1600 John F. Kennedy Boulevard • Suite 1800 • Philadelphia, Pennsylvania, 19103-2899

http://www.theclinics.com

IMMUNOLOGY AND ALLERGY CLINICS OF NORTH AMERICA Volume 37, Number 3

August 2017 ISSN 0889-8561, ISBN-13: 978-0-323-53237-2

Editor: Jessica McCool

Developmental Editor: Kristen Helm

Immunology and Allergy Clinics of North America (ISSN 0889–8561) is published quarterly by Elsevier Inc., 360 Park Avenue South, New York, NY 10010-1710. Months of issue are February, May, August, and November. Periodicals postage paid at New York, NY and additional mailing offices. Subscription prices are $320.00 per year for US individuals, $528.00 per year for US institutions, $100.00 per year for US students and residents, $395.00 per year for Canadian individuals, $220.00 per year for Canadian students, $670.00 per year for Canadian institutions, $445.00 per year for international individuals, $670.00 per year for international institutions, $220.00 per year for international students. To receive student/resident rate, orders must be accompanied by name of affiliated institution, date of term, and the *signature* of program/residency coordinator on institution letterhead. Orders will be billed at individual rate until proof of status is received. Foreign air speed delivery is included in all *Clinics* subscription prices. All prices are subject to change without notice. **POSTMASTER:** Send address changes to *Immunology and Allergy Clinics of North America*, Elsevier Health Sciences Division, Subscription Customer Service, 3251 Riverport Lane, Maryland Heights, MO 63043. **Customer Service: 1-800-654-2452 (U.S. and Canada); 314-447-8871 (outside U.S. and Canada). Fax: 314-447-8029. E-mail: journalscustomerservice-usa@elsevier.com** (for print support); **journalsonlinesupport-usa@elsevier.com (for online support).**

Reprints. For copies of 100 or more, of articles in this publication, please contact the Commercial Reprints Department, Elsevier Inc., 360 Park Avenue South, New York, New York 10010-1710. Tel. 212-633-3874, Fax: 212-633-3820, E-mail: reprints@elsevier.com.

Immunology and Allergy Clinics of North America is covered in MEDLINE/PubMed (Index Medicus), Current Contents/Life Sciences, Science Citation Index, ISI/BIOMED, Chemical Abstracts, and EMBASE/Excerpta Medica.

Contributors

CONSULTING EDITOR

STEPHEN A. TILLES, MD
Executive Director, ASTHMA Inc. Clinical Research Center, Partner, Northwest Asthma and Allergy Center, Clinical Professor of Medicine, University of Washington, Seattle, Washington

EDITOR

MARC A. RIEDL, MD, MS
Professor of Medicine, Clinical Director, US HAEA Angioedema Center, Training Program Director, Division of Rheumatology, Allergy and Immunology, Department of Medicine, University of California, San Diego, La Jolla, California

AUTHORS

ALEENA BANERJI, MD
Division of Rheumatology, Allergy and Immunology, Department of Medicine, Massachusetts General Hospital, Boston, Massachusetts

STEPHEN D. BETSCHEL, MD, FRCPC
Division of Clinical Immunology, St Michael's Hospital, University of Toronto, Toronto, Ontario, Canada

NANCY J. BROWN, MD
Chair, Department of Medicine, Physician-in-Chief, Hugh J. Morgan Professor of Medicine and Pharmacology, Vanderbilt University Medical Center, Nashville, Tennessee

PAULA J. BUSSE, MD
Associate Professor, Division of Allergy and Clinical Immunology, Icahn School of Medicine at Mount Sinai, New York, New York

TERESA CABALLERO, MD, PhD
Allergy Department, Hospital La Paz Institute for Health Research, CIBERER, Madrid, Spain

MENG CHEN, MD
Division of Rheumatology, Allergy and Immunology, Department of Medicine, University of California, San Diego, San Diego, California

SANDRA C. CHRISTIANSEN, MD
Department of Medicine, University of California, San Diego, La Jolla, California

ANASTASIOS E. GERMENIS, MD, PhD
Department of Immunology and Histocompatibility, Faculty of Medicine, School of Health Sciences, University of Thessaly, Larissa, Greece

PARWINDER GILL, MD, FRCPC, ABIM
Division of Clinical Immunology and Allergy, St Joseph's Hospital, Western University, London, Ontario, Canada

KUSUMAM JOSEPH, PhD
Department of Biochemistry and Molecular Biology, Medical University of South Carolina, Charleston, South Carolina

ALLEN P. KAPLAN, MD
Department of Medicine, Medical University of South Carolina, Charleston, South Carolina

CONSTANCE H. KATELARIS, MD, PhD, FRACP
Professor, Immunology and Allergy Unit, Department of Medicine, Head of Unit, Campbelltown Hospital, Sydney, New South Wales, Australia

HILARY LONGHURST, MA, FRCP, PhD, FRCPath
Consultant Immunologist, Department of Immunology, Barts Health NHS Trust, London, United Kingdom

WILLIAM R. LUMRY, MD
Clinical Professor, Internal Medicine/Allergy/Immunology Division, University of Texas Southwestern Medical School, Medical Director, AARA Research Associates, Private Practice, Dallas, Texas

COEN MAAS, PhD
Department of Clinical Chemistry and Haematology, University Medical Center Utrecht, Utrecht, The Netherlands

MARKUS MAGERL, MD
Professor of Dermatology and Allergy, Department of Dermatology and Allergy, Allergie-Centrum-Charité/ECARF, Charité - Universitätsmedizin Berlin, Berlin, Germany

MARCUS MAURER, MD
Professor of Dermatology and Allergy, Department of Dermatology and Allergy, Allergie-Centrum-Charité /ECARF, Charité - Universitätsmedizin Berlin, Berlin, Germany

IRIS M. OTANI, MD
Division of Pulmonary, Allergy, Critical Care, and Sleep Medicine, Department of Medicine, Univeristy of California San Francisco Medical Center, San Francisco, California

NIEVES PRIOR, MD, PhD
Allergy Department, Hospital Universitario Severo Ochoa, Leganés, Madrid, Spain

MARC A. RIEDL, MD, MS
Professor of Medicine, Clinical Director, US HAEA Angioedema Center, Training Program Director, Division of Rheumatology, Allergy and Immunology, Department of Medicine, University of California, San Diego, La Jolla, California

TUKISA SMITH, MD
Clinical Fellow, Division of Allergy and Clinical Immunology, Icahn School of Medicine at Mount Sinai, New York, New York

COSBY STONE Jr, MD, MPH
Post-Doctoral Research Fellow in Allergy and Immunology, Division of Allergy, Pulmonary and Critical Care Medicine, Vanderbilt University Medical Center, Nashville, Tennessee

EMILY ZINSER, MA, MBBS, MRCP
Specialty Registrar in Immunology, Department of Immunology, Barts Health NHS Trust, London, United Kingdom

BRUCE L. ZURAW, MD
Department of Medicine, University of California, San Diego, La Jolla, San Diego Veterans Administration Healthcare System, San Diego, California

Contents

Acquired angioedema due to C1-INH deficiency (C1-INH-AAE) can occur when there are acquired (not inherited) deficiencies of C1-INH. A quantitative or functional C1-INH deficiency with negative family history and low C1q is diagnostic of C1-INH-AAE. The most common conditions associated with C1-INH-AAE are autoimmunity and B-cell lymphoproliferative disorders. A diagnosis of C1-INH-AAE can precede a diagnosis of lymphoproliferative disease and confers an increased risk for developing non-Hodgkin lymphoma. Treatment focuses on symptom control with therapies that regulate bradykinin activity (C1-INH concentrate, icatibant, ecallantide, tranexamic acid, androgens) and treatment of any underlying conditions.

Hereditary angioedema (HAE) is an autosomal-dominant disorder owing to mutations in the C1 inhibitor gene. Type I is characterized by a low C1 inhibitor protein level and diminished functional activity, whereas type II has a normal (or elevated) protein level but diminished function. When functional levels drop beyond 40% of normal, attacks of swelling are likely to occur due to overproduction of bradykinin. Angioedema can be peripheral, abdominal, or laryngeal. The typical duration of episodes is 3 days. Therapies include C1 inhibitor replacement for prophylaxis or acute therapy, whereas inhibition of kallikrein or blockade at the bradykinin receptor level can interrupt acute episodes of swelling.

Hereditary angioedema (HAE) is a rare autosomal dominant disease clinically characterized by recurrent, often unpredictable attacks of subcutaneous and mucosal swelling. Acute episodes are debilitating, painful, disfiguring, and potentially fatal. HAE type I and type II result from a deficiency in the plasma level of functional C1 inhibitor. HAE with normal levels of C1 inhibitor has been recognized. There is evidence that contact activation underlies the recurrent attacks of swelling. This article reviews laboratory parameters to detect contact system activation and implications for diagnosis of HAE and other forms of bradykinin-mediated angioedema.

Several treatment modalities have become available for management of acute hereditary angioedema (HAE) attacks in the last 15 years. Most are now available to patients in North America, Europe, United Kingdom, and Australia, but few options exist in developing countries. Preferred contemporary use of the treatments to be discussed is "on demand," because control remains with the patient and delays in treatment access avoided. Four treatments—plasma-derived C1 inhibitor concentrate, recombinant C1 inhibitor concentrate, ecallantide, and icatibant—are reviewed in this article. All have been shown to be superior to placebo and effective in the management of all HAE attacks.

Hilary Longhurst and Emily Zinser

Long-term prophylaxis is needed in many patients with hereditary angioedema and poses many challenges. Attenuated androgens are effective in many but are limited by side effect profiles. There is less evidence for efficacy of tranexamic acid and progestagens; however, the small side effect profile makes tranexamic acid an option for prophylaxis in children and progestagens an option for women. C1 inhibitor is beneficial, but at present requires intravenous delivery and may need dose titration for maximum efficacy. Short-term prophylaxis should be considered for all procedures. New therapies are promising in overcoming many problems encountered with current options for long-term prophylaxis.

Markus Magerl, Anastasios E. Germenis, Coen Maas, and Marcus Maurer

A new form of hereditary angioedema (HAE) was identified in the year 2000. Its clinical appearance resembles HAE types I and II, which are caused by mutations that result in low levels of C1 inhibitor (C1-INH). In patients with this form of HAE, C1-INH plasma levels and function values are normal, so it is termed HAE with normal C1-INH (HAE-nC1). HAE-nC1, in a subgroup of patients, is thought to be caused by mutations that affect the F12 gene. The diagnosis of HAE-nC1 is based on history and clinical criteria. There are no licensed drugs with proven treatment effects for HAE-nC1.

Meng Chen and Marc A. Riedl

Remarkable progress has been made in the treatment of bradykinin-mediated angioedema with the advent of multiple new therapies. Patients now have effective medications available for prophylaxis and treatment of acute attacks. However, hereditary angioedema is a burdensome disease that can lead to debilitating and dangerous angioedema episodes associated with significant costs for individuals and society. The burden of treatment must be addressed regarding medication administration difficulties, treatment complications, and adverse side effects. New therapies are being investigated and may offer solutions to these challenges. This article reviews the emerging therapeutic options for the treatment of HAE.

Teresa Caballero and Nieves Prior

Burden of illness studies and evaluation of health-related quality of life using validated questionnaires have become an important task in the comprehensive management of angioedema conditions, mainly angioedema associated with chronic spontaneous urticaria and hereditary angioedema caused by C1-inhibitor deficiency. A review of the principal tools and studies is presented. Both diseases present a higher proportion of psychiatric disorders, impair work and studies productivity, and produce high direct and indirect costs. These assessments also have been useful to evaluate the positive impact of new drugs and interventions. More studies are desirable, especially in other types of angioedema disorders, such as hereditary angioedema with normal C1 inhibitor.

This article discusses orphan diseases, their prevalence, legislative incentives to encourage development of therapies, and the impact of treatment on health care payment systems. Specifically, the cost burden of hereditary angioedema on patients, health care systems, and society is reviewed. The impact of availability of and access to novel and specific therapies on morbidity, mortality, and overall burden of disease is explored. Changes in treatment paradigms to improve effect and reduce cost of treatment are presented.

IMMUNOLOGY AND ALLERGY CLINICS OF NORTH AMERICA

THE CLINICS ARE AVAILABLE ONLINE!
Access your subscription at:
www.theclinics.com

Foreword

Angioedema: An Orphan Symptom with Its Own Orphan Disease

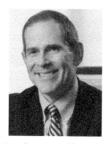

Stephen A. Tilles, MD
Consulting Editor

Angioedema is a common symptom encountered by allergy/immunology specialists in everyday practice, though it is only rarely the overriding reason for a doctor visit. In its most common form, angioedema is histamine mediated and occurs concurrently with urticaria. Patients often focus much more on the urticaria, mentioning angioedema more as an afterthought. However, at other times angioedema involves acute disfiguring of the lips, eyelids, and other parts of the face to the point that the patient becomes unrecognizable. Worse yet, on very rare occasions, angioedema of the larynx results in catastrophic upper airway obstruction and asphyxiation.

Determining whether angioedema without concurrent urticaria is mediated by histamine has emerged in recent years as a key decision point with critical implications regarding likely cause and management strategy. Bradykinin is the other main mediator of angioedema, as its overproduction results in increased endothelial cell permeability resulting in angioedema without urticaria. This category of angioedema is much less common than histamine-mediated angioedema, as the main disease in this category, hereditary angioedema (HAE), affects fewer than 10,000 patients in the United States. However, HAE is permanent, recurrent, and often debilitating, and therefore, the recent emergence of effective therapeutics for bradykinin-induced angioedema has dramatically improved the lives of many patients.

This issue of *Immunology and Allergy Clinics of North America* takes on the broad subject of angioedema, including both histamine-mediated and bradykinin-mediated forms. Guest Editor Marc Riedl has assembled an impressive group of prominent authors to summarize a variety of relevant topics, including clinical evaluation, an overview of angioedema mediated by histamine, ACE inhibitor–induced angioedema, acquired C1 inhibitor deficiency, and several reviews that address HAE, including

Immunol Allergy Clin N Am 37 (2017) xiii–xiv
http://dx.doi.org/10.1016/j.iac.2017.05.002
0889-8561/17/© 2017 Published by Elsevier Inc.

one that focuses on the pharmacoeconomics of orphan disease drug development. This issue is a valuable reference for practicing allergy/immunology specialists and other providers who encounter angioedema patients in their practices.

Stephen A. Tilles, MD
ASTHMA Inc. Clinical Research Center
Northwest Asthma and Allergy Center
University of Washington
9725 3rd Avenue Northeast, Suite 500
Seattle, WA 98115, USA

E-mail address:
stilles@nwasthma.com

Preface

Angioedema: Challenges and Insights

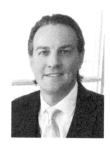

Marc A. Riedl, MD, MS
Editor

Angioedema remains a challenging and vexing condition confronting a variety of medical specialists. While reasonably common within the general population, the wide variability in clinical presentation, severity, and underlying causes can lead to considerable frustration for the affected individual as well as health care professionals assessing the patient. This issue of *Immunology and Allergy Clinics of North America* aims to provide a useful guide for clinical practice through a comprehensive review of angioedema conditions provided by leading experts in the field.

Parwinder Gill and Stephen Betschel provide a comprehensive overview of the angioedema evaluation, including the differential diagnosis, clinical considerations, and useful laboratory assessment. Frequently in clinical practice, initial evaluation will suggest a histamine-mediated angioedema condition prompting a more specific course of evaluation and treatment. Paula Busse and Tukisa Smith review this area of angioedema in their article. A critical aspect of the clinical evaluation is consideration of medication-induced angioedema, as ACE-I and other medications account for a substantial portion of events seen in the acute or emergency setting. Cosby Stone Jr and Nancy Brown provide an update on the current understanding of medication-related angioedema. Less common causes of angioedema may be overlooked or misdiagnosed in clinical practice, leading to diagnostic delays, ineffective therapy, and subsequent complications, particularly given the potential severity of these rarer conditions. Iris Otani and Aleena Banerji review acquired C1INH deficiency in the fourth article, while Allen Kaplan and Kusumam Joseph contribute a detailed discussion of the pathophysiology of hereditary angioedema (HAE). A continuing major challenge within the angioedema field is the limited diagnostic biomarkers available. Sandra Christiansen and Bruce Zuraw provide an update on laboratory approaches to evaluating the contact system in their article in this issue. With advances in medical therapy, the clinical management of HAE has changed remarkably over the past decade in many parts

Immunol Allergy Clin N Am 37 (2017) xv–xvi
http://dx.doi.org/10.1016/j.iac.2017.05.001
0889-8561/17/© 2017 Published by Elsevier Inc.   immunology.theclinics.com

of the world. To address this, Constance Katelaris reviews the current state of acute treatment for HAE, while Hilary Longhurst and Emily Zinser summarize prophylactic approaches to managing HAE. As perhaps the "newest" recognized angioedema condition, HAE with normal C1INH remains an area of intense investigation. Markus Magerl, Anastasios E. Germenis, Coen Maas, and Marcus Maurer review the latest advances in understanding and managing HAE with normal C1INH inhibitor. Looking toward the future, Meng Chen and Marc Riedl review the most recent developments in angioedema therapeutics with a focus on investigational agents that may impact the current treatment paradigm. Teresa Caballero and Nieves Prior provide a thorough review of the current data on burden of illness and quality of life related to angioedema conditions in their article. William Lumry concludes the issue with a review of pharmacoeconomic considerations in the management of rare conditions, with a specific discussion of HAE.

With this issue, I believe the authors have addressed the most challenging and fascinating aspects of the angioedema universe. I wish to thank each of them for their tremendous efforts in developing these excellent focused reviews, and I expect their articles will be valuable to colleagues called upon to evaluate and manage individuals affected by angioedema symptoms. Most importantly, I hope the information within these articles will lead to better lives for patients and improved outcomes for health care systems while stimulating additional research progress within the field.

Marc A. Riedl, MD, MS
US HAEA Angioedema Center
Allergy & Immunology
University of California, San Diego
8899 University Center Lane, Suite 230
La Jolla, CA 92122, USA

E-mail address:
mriedl@ucsd.edu

The Clinical Evaluation of Angioedema

Parwinder Gill, MD, FRCPC, ABIM[a], Stephen D. Betschel, MD, FRCPC[b],*

KEYWORDS

- Angioedema • Bradykinin • Histamine • Hereditary angioedema

KEY POINTS

- Angioedema may occur through several mechanistic pathways. An understanding of the pathophysiology aids in the evaluation, clinical diagnosis, and management of this condition.
- Angioedema can be broadly categorized into episodes occurring with or without urticaria; after this distinction is made, this allows for the further differentiation of angioedema subtypes.
- The initial step in the clinical evaluation of angioedema is obtaining a thorough patient and family history, while giving consideration to differential diagnoses and angioedema mimickers.
- Although episodes of angioedema without urticaria may be clinically similar in presentation, there are characteristics and laboratory parameters that are unique to each subtype. Applying an algorithmic approach based on these parameters allows one to reach an accurate diagnosis.
- Further research in the clinical evaluation of angioedema directed at developing a greater understanding of the pathophysiology should enable the development of new diagnostic assays and novel targeted treatments.

INTRODUCTION

Angioedema, also known as Quincke edema or "angioneurotic edema," was first described by Marcello Donati in 1586 in reference to a young count who developed lip swelling as a result of an egg allergy.[1] The first reference to hereditary angioedema resulting in fatal suffocation was reported by Osler in 1885.[2]

It is estimated that up to 25% of the US population will experience an episode of urticaria with or without angioedema during their lifetime.[3] Angioedema is defined

Disclosure Statement: P. Gill has no disclosures relevant to this publication. S.D. Betschel has received research funding from CSL Behring and advisory fees from Shire and CSL-Behring.
a Division of Clinical Immunology, St. Joseph's Hospital, Western University, 268 Grosvenor Street, London, ON N6A 4V2, Canada; b Division of Clinical Immunology and Allergy, St. Michael's Hospital, 30 Bond Street, Toronto, ON M5B 1W8, Canada
* Corresponding author.
E-mail address: BetschelS@smh.ca

as the localized nonpitting edema of deep dermal, subcutaneous, or submucosal tissues resulting from the increase in vascular permeability and extravasation of intravascular fluids; although it can coincide with urticaria in a histamine-mediated process, a differentiating feature is that urticarial wheals are limited to the mid and papillary dermis.[3]

This article serves as a general overview of the clinical evaluation of angioedema with and without urticaria and focuses on the following:

1. Signs and symptoms of angioedema
2. Classification of angioedema subtypes
3. Pathophysiology
4. An approach to the clinical evaluation of angioedema
5. Diagnostic evaluation in angioedema
6. Future directions in the evaluation of angioedema

More detailed discussion about angioedema mechanisms and treatments will be presented in other sections of this issue of *Immunology and Allergy Clinics of North America*.

SIGNS AND SYMPTOMS OF ANGIOEDEMA

The presentation of angioedema may vary between subtypes, although in all forms, it can occur at any site of the body and some organ tissues. The edema itself is nonpitting, typically with ill-defined borders, and may be flesh-colored or erythematous in nature. Episodes of swelling may be accompanied by pruritus and urticaria, in the case of histamine-mediated forms, or associated with a burning and tingling sensation.

The most commonly involved sites include the following:

1. Head and neck: Angioedema affecting the eyelids, lips, tongue, and larynx, with the possibility of life-threatening airway obstruction
2. Peripheries: Swelling of the hands, feet, and urogenital areas
3. Abdomen: Angioedema may mimic symptoms of an acute abdomen, resulting in surgical intervention

Examples of these site-specific swellings are depicted in **Fig. 1** and **Fig. 2**.

Several factors are known to increase the probability as well as the severity of specific angioedema subtypes as discussed later, but can include foods and medications resulting in direct mast cell degranulation (ie alcohol, non-steroidal anti-inflammatory drugs [NSAIDs]), stress, dental or surgical manipulation, and hormonal factors.[4,5]

PATHOPHYSIOLOGY OF ANGIOEDEMA

Acute episodes of angioedema result from a release of vasoactive mediators that increase vascular permeability in the skin and submucosa, allowing for the vascular leakage of plasma and resultant edema; most of these attacks can be attributable to the following.

Histamine-Mediated Pathways

Immunoglobulin E (IgE)-mediated reaction begins with a primary response and typically occurs within seconds to minutes of exposure to an allergen, from the release of vasoactive amines such as histamine, and results in increased vascular permeability, smooth muscle contraction, vasodilation, glandular secretions, and bronchospasm.[6]

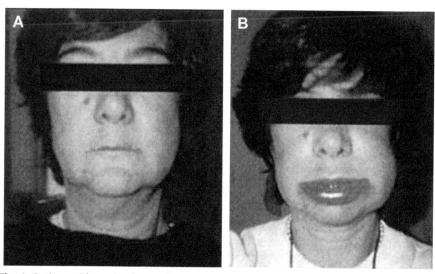

Fig. 1. Patient with angioedema affecting her lips: a comparison between (*A*) baseline and (*B*) during an attack. (*Adapted from* Bowen T, Cicardi M, Farkas H, et al. Canadian 2003 International Consensus Algorithm for the diagnosis, therapy, and management of hereditary angioedema. J Allergy Clin Immunol 2004;114(3):631; with permission.)

The secondary, or late phase response, occurs 8 to 12 hours after allergen exposure and results from the synthesis of leukotrienes, chemokines, prostaglandins, and platelet-activating factor (**Fig. 3**).[7] The late phase response results in tissue infiltration by leukocytes, specifically eosinophils, resulting in an inflammatory response and the production of leukotrienes and prostaglandins.[6]

There may be an association with autoantibodies directed against the Fc-epsilon receptor (FcεR) of both the mast cell and the IgE molecules, resulting in histamine release and the development of urticaria and angioedema.[8] The high-affinity form of this receptor, FcεR1, plays a significant role in allergic diseases, in addition to the production of inflammatory mediators.[9] This mechanism can be demonstrated through the use of an autologous serum skin test, where the intradermal injection of one's own serum results in a wheal and flare response.[10]

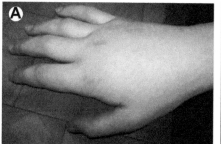
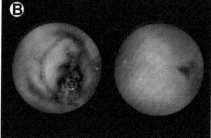

Fig. 2. (*A*) Angioedema of the hand in a patient with hereditary angioedema. (*B*) Capsule endoscopy during abdominal attack in patient with hereditary angioedema, showing ileal tract with normal mucosa and lumen (*left*), and edematous ileum and substantially reduced luminal diameter, causing partial bowel obstruction (*right*). (*From* Longhurst H, Cicardi M. Hereditary angio-oedema. Lancet 2012;379(9814):475; with permission.)

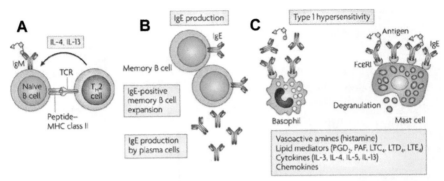

Fig. 3. (*A*) TH2 cell interaction with naive B cells leads to immunoglobulin class switch to IgE and expansion of allergen-specific memory B cells. (*B*) IgE produced by plasma cells sensitizes mast cells and basophils by binding to surface FcRI. (*C*) The crosslinking of basophil and mast-cell surface FcRI-bound IgE by B-cell epitopes of allergens leads to the release of vasoactive amines (such as histamine), lipid mediators (such as prostaglandin D2 [PGD2], platelet-activating factor [PAF], leukotriene [LT] C4 [LTC4], LTD4 and LTE4, cytokines and chemokines), and to the immediate symptoms of allergic disease (type I hypersensitivity), including pruritus, wheal and flare, nasal conjunctival discharge, angioedema, systemic anaphylaxis, and bronchoconstriction. T-regulatory (TReg) cells modulate type-1 hypersensitivity reactions by suppression of IgE and induction of blocking antibodies by interleukin-10 (IL-10), suppression of mast-cell tissue infiltration by IL-10 and transforming growth factor (TGF), and suppression of TH2 cells by IL-10 and TGFβ. MHC, major histocompatibility complex; TCR, T-cell receptor. (*From* Akdis M, Akdis CA. Therapeutic manipulation of immune tolerance in allergic disease. Nat Rev Drug Discov 2009;8(8):650; with permission.)

Bradykinin-Mediated Pathways

In the case of hereditary, acquired, or angiotensin-converting enzyme inhibitor (ACE inhibitor) -induced angioedema, the vasodilatory peptide, bradykinin, plays a key role in endothelial cell activation, with resultant tissue edema.[11] Bradykinin is released from many cell types, and mechanisms that interfere in either its production, or as in the case of ACE inhibitors, its degradation, result in angioedema.

Angioedema may occur through several mechanisms as outlined in later discussion, namely, the complement, coagulation, and contact pathways that are essential in the regulation of bradykinin.

C1-esterase inhibitor (C1-INH) is a member of the serine protease family (serpin), whose role it is to prevent the formation of the C1 complex and the consequent complement activation. It also acts as a direct inhibitor of activated kallikrein.[11] C1-INH also plays a regulatory role in fibrinolytic, coagulation, and kinin pathways.[12]

In hereditary angioedema type 1 and 2 (HAE-1 and HAE-2), there is a deficiency in an inhibitory enzyme of the complement system, C1-INH, which results in complement activation and kallikrein production, both contributing to the production of bradykinin (**Fig. 4**).[13] C1-INH deficiencies also affect the complement pathway, fibrinolytic system, and the intrinsic coagulation pathways.

Mutations in the SERPING1 gene located on the eleventh chromosome result in decreased antigenic levels of C1-INH seen in HAE-1 or a functional impairment, as in HAE-2.[4] Both are inherited in an autosomal dominant manner, although up to 25% of all cases may be due to spontaneous mutations.[14–16] HAE-1 occurs in 86% of cases,[16] whereas HAE-2 is less commonly identified (in up to 15% of cases); HAE-nC1INH is inherited in an autosomal dominant manner and occurs mostly in

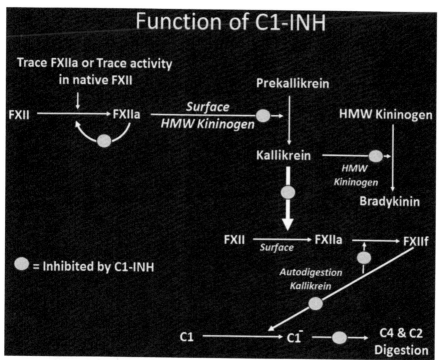

Fig. 4. Zinc-dependent binding of factor XII and HK to vascular endothelial cells. Although both bind to gC1qR, which is present in excess, there is preferential binding of factor XII to the complex of u-PAR and cytokeratin 1, while HK binds primarily to the complex of gC1qR and cytokeratin 1. HK, high-molecular-weight kininogen.

women. However, some male patients have been reported. In some cases, HAE-nC-INH may be associated with a gain of function mutation in Factor XII, resulting in kinin overproduction.[14]

Investigations into the role of the coagulation and contact pathway in angioedema have found that dysregulation of these processes may result in increased clotting activities of Factors XII, XI, and V. An in vitro diagnostic test, activated partial thromboplastin time (APTT), can be used as a surrogate marker of both the intrinsic and common coagulation pathways and the contact system. Recent research has shown that shortened APTT levels are seen in individuals with deficient levels and function of the C1-INH as well as in acquired forms of angioedema in comparison to angioedema with normal C1-INH.[17]

In the case of HAE-1, it is the level and function of C1-INH that are decreased, whereas in HAE-2, there is a normal level of C1-INH, but a functional deficiency. The pathophysiology of HAE-nC1INH is poorly understood, because there are no detectable abnormalities in the C1-INH, but has been associated with mutations in the Factor XII gene. Acquired causes of bradykinin-mediated angioedema have been associated with antibody production against the C1-inhibitor enzyme itself.[6,11]

Further insights into the pathophysiology and mechanisms underlying these processes are addressed in later sections of this issue of *Immunology and Allergy Clinics of North America*, which are devoted to hereditary angioedema.

Angioedema Resulting Through Cyclooxygenase 1 Inhibition

Angioedema may arise as a consequence of the inhibition of cyclooxygenase 1 (COX-1), leading to unopposed arachidonic metabolism, with resultant leukotriene synthesis, as by NSAIDs. The net result of the accumulation of these vasoactive cysteinyl leukotrienes is an increase in vascular permeability, fluid extravasation, and resultant edema.[18]

Type III Hypersensitivity Reactions

A rarer cause of angioedema and urticaria results from the formation of antigen-antibody complexes through type III hypersensitivity reactions (as in the case of urticarial vasculitis).[19]

Table 1 summarizes the key differences in pathophysiologic mechanisms of angioedema subtypes.[18,20,21]

CLASSIFICATION OF ANGIOEDEMA

The most common form of angioedema is the allergic type, followed by idiopathic and ACE-inhibitor induced. Hereditary and acquired forms are relatively rare in comparison.[14] Angioedema can be classified into several subtypes, differentiated by the clinical presentation and pathophysiology:

1. Histaminergic (through IgE-independent or -dependent mechanisms)
2. Idiopathic
3. Hereditary angioedema (HAE-1, HAE-2, and HAE-nC1INH)
4. Acquired angioedema (including ACEi-induced and C1-INH deficiency)

APPROACH TO THE CLINICAL EVALUATION AND DIAGNOSTIC WORKUP

In addition to obtaining a thorough patient and family history of angioedema, the clinical presentation, time to the onset of symptoms, and recognition of differentiating characteristics are imperative in making an accurate diagnosis.

Histamine-Mediated Angioedema

Clinical features

Allergic angioedema The initial stratification of angioedema subtypes involves determining if these attacks are accompanied by pruritic urticarial wheals, which can be categorized as histamine-mediated or "allergic" angioedema, resulting from mast cell degranulation and the release of inflammatory mediators such as histamine in either IgE-dependent or -independent manners. Triggers may include foods, medications, latex, insect bites, and stings, for example.

In addition to angioedema, these reactions can manifest with a combination of one or more symptoms involving the respiratory, cardiac, neurologic, or gastrointestinal systems.[3] Symptoms may include wheezing, coughing, chest pain or tightness, nausea, vomiting, lightheadedness, and even shock as a result of hypotension.

A differentiating feature of this form of angioedema is that it responds to treatment with corticosteroids, epinephrine, and antihistamines. Symptoms tend to be of shorter duration (typically <24 hours).[3] Nonallergic forms of angioedema tend to worsen over the course of 24 to 36 hours and may last up to 3 to 5 days without appropriate treatment.[13] Histaminergic angioedema can occur at various sites in the body, although in comparison to non-histamine-mediated forms of angioedema, it less commonly involves the genitalia.[3]

Table 1
Molecular mechanisms of angioedema

Type of AE	Mediator	Mechanism
Allergic AE	Histamine (mast cells)	Allergens react with IgE antibodies on the surface of mast cells, causing degranulation and release of histamine
ACE-I-induced	Bradykinin	ACE-Is prevent the conversion of bradykinin to inactive metabolites, leading to bradykinin accumulation
NSAID-induced AE	Leukotrienes (mast cells)	Inhibition of COX-1 leads to overproduction of vasoactive substances by shunting arachidonic acid metabolism through the lipoxygenase pathway, creating leukotrienes; vasoactive leukotrienes act on cell-surface receptors to increase vascular permeability and promote inflammation
HAE type 1	Bradykinin	Genetic mutations in the *C1 INH* gene result in low levels of C1 INH; major roles of C1 INH include inactivating coagulation factors XIIa. XIIf and XIa: blocking C1 complement autoactivation and inhibiting activated kallikrein; removal of these inhibitory actions results in complement activation and elevated bradykinin levels
HAE type 2	Bradykinin	Genetic mutations in the *C1 INH* gene result in normal levels of C1INH, but the C1 INH is dysfunctional; plasma cascades are unregulated in the presence of dysfunctional C1 INH, leading to bradykinin accumulation as in HAE type 1
Inherited AE with normal C1 INH	Bradykinin	Missense mutation in factor XII gene confers a significant increase in the protease activity of each activated factor XII molecule, which increases bradykinin generation; decreased activity of enzymes such as ACE and aminopeptidase P have also been noted
Acquired AE	Bradykinin	Type 1: Immune complex formation associated with rheumatologic, lymphoproliferative, and neoplastic disorders continuously activate C1, causing C1 INH depletion and bradykinin accumulation Type 2: Autoantibodies inactivate C1 INH, leading to bradykinin accumulation
Idiopathic recurrent AE	Unknown	Unknown

Abbreviation: AE, adverse events.

From Nzeako UC. Diagnosis and management of angioedema with abdominal involvement: a gastroenterology perspective. World J Gastroenterol 2010;16(39):4914; with permission.

Pseudoallergic angioedema Angioedema (with or without urticaria) developing after the use of NSAIDs may be either "pseudoallergic" or IgE mediated. Several subtypes of angioedema and urticaria with NSAID use have been identified[22]:

1. NSAID-exacerbated angioedema or urticaria in up to 10% to 30% of those with underlying chronic urticaria.[23]
2. NSAID-induced angioedema or urticaria in individuals without chronic urticaria.
3. Single NSAID-induced angioedema, urticaria, or anaphylaxis occurring in an IgE-dependent manner; these individuals may react to structurally related NSAIDs as well.

Idiopathic angioedema In a significant number of patients, no identifiable cause is found for recurrent episodes of angioedema with or without urticaria and is deemed as "idiopathic" in nature once alternate identifiable causes have been excluded.[24] Idiopathic cases may occur in antibody-dependent and -independent mechanisms and typically respond to antihistamines and corticosteroids.[14]

In a study conducted by Zingale and colleagues[24] evaluating angioedema without urticaria, a specific cause was found in 16% of all patients (n = 776), and most of the cases were attributed to drugs, foods, and stings. Furthermore, in 7% of cases, an underlying disease process or infection was identified. ACE inhibitors contributed to 11% of all reactions, with a median time to onset of symptoms at 12 months after initiating therapy.[24–26] Hence, it is important to evaluate for an underlying cause of angioedema before calling it idiopathic.

Consideration should be given to rare causes of angioedema if there is concern of an underlying autoimmune condition, malignancy, or inflammatory condition because the evaluation may require additional testing. Similarly, if the patient's history and clinical presentation are atypical of either a histaminergic- or bradykinin-mediated process, one must rule out common mimickers.

DIAGNOSTIC EVALUATION OF HISTAMINE-MEDIATED ANGIOEDEMA

In cases of "allergic" and "pseudoallergic" angioedema, the clinical history aids in determining whether further diagnostic testing is required. In the case of specific triggers, such as foods, medications, bites or stings, skin prick testing, the use of specific IgE measurements, and oral challenges to foods and medications may be useful in identifying the culprit. A serum tryptase level and urine histamine levels are useful markers in that they may be elevated in acute episodes of histamine-mediated angioedema and urticaria.[3] To note, in histaminergic angioedema, serum complement levels as well as C1-INH antigenic and functional levels are unaffected.

There are several additional investigations that may be useful in the evaluation of angioedema, both with and without urticaria. Investigations should be geared toward differential diagnoses and mimickers and may be useful in the workup of idiopathic or acquired forms of angioedema (**Table 2**).

If an underlying hematologic cause such as multiple myeloma or malignancy is of concern, a complete blood count with smear and differential may identify cytopenias, and a serum protein electrophoresis with immunofixation can be used to identify clonal immunoglobulin populations. A targeted malignancy workup (ie with imaging and biopsies) can also be pursued if there are organ-specific symptoms.

If autoimmunity or an inflammatory process is suspected, screening tests to consider would include an antinuclear antibody (ANA), rheumatoid factor, and inflammatory markers such as erythrocyte sedimentation rate (ESR), C-reactive protein (CRP), ferritin, all of which may be elevated in these conditions. Furthermore, positive thyroid antibodies have been shown to be associated with chronic spontaneous urticaria, although their significance in the disease process is not well established.

In cases of immunodeficiencies associated with urticaria or angioedema, such as Gleich syndrome presenting with elevated IgM, angioedema and eosinophilia, quantitative immunoglobulins (IgA, IgG, and IgM), CH50, C3 levels, and immunoassays can be considered.

In ruling out angioedema mimickers related to infectious processes such as cellulitis, consideration may be given to obtaining blood and tissue cultures, in addition to skin biopsies. As peripheral edema secondary to impairments in the circulatory or lymphatic symptoms may resemble angioedema, electrolytes including renal function and a urinalysis may be helpful in identifying hypoalbuminemia and proteinuria.

Table 2
Summary of additional investigations to consider in the workup of acquired and idiopathic angioedema

Diagnostic Test	Significance
Specific IgE levels, skin prick testing, and oral challenges to suspected foods/medications	To evaluate for IgE-mediated causes of urticaria and angioedema
Serum tryptase and urine histamine	To evaluate for histaminergic causes of urticaria and angioedema
Complete blood count with smear and differential	To evaluate for cytopenias and hematologic malignancies
Serum protein electrophoresis with immunofixation	To evaluate for clonal populations, such as in multiple myeloma
Targeted malignancy workup	In the case of idiopathic or acquired forms
Quantitative immunoglobulins (IgG, IgA, IgM)	To evaluate for immunodeficiencies and conditions associated with urticaria and angioedema (ie, Gleich syndrome with elevated IgM, angioedema, and eosinophilia)
CH50, C3, and immune complex assays	To screen for associated complement deficiencies
Inflammatory and autoimmune markers: ESR, CRP, ferritin, rheumatoid factor, ANA	May be elevated in the case of autoimmune causes or inflammatory conditions
Thyroid function and antibodies	Associated with chronic spontaneous urticaria and autoimmune disease
Cultures (blood, tissue, throat, and urine) and infectious workup	To rule out infection or cellulitis as a mimicker or cause
Urinalysis and electrolytes	May identify proteinuria and hypoalbuminemia as causes of edema

During acute attacks, if organ involvement is considered, imaging studies such as radiographs, ultrasounds, and computed tomographic scans may be useful in identifying soft tissue swelling of the neck, ascites, and edema of the gastrointestinal tract.[27]

If no confirmatory diagnosis can be made on the basis of these investigations, a trial of empiric therapy with antihistamines, corticosteroids, and epinephrine can be considered in the evaluation of histaminergic angioedema.

Bradykinin-Mediated Angioedema

Clinical features

Hereditary angioedema Hereditary angioedema is estimated to affect 1 in 10,000 to 1 in 50,000 individuals.[28] Patients may present with angioedema affecting many organ systems in an asymmetric distribution, including involvement of the head and neck, with concerns of life-threatening laryngeal attacks that may result in asphyxiation as well as swelling of peripheral tissues, urogenital edema, and abdominal pain. In up to 50% of cases, these attacks may be preceded by a tingling sensation or erythema marginatum, with nonpitting angioedema that is nonpruritic in nature.[3]

The severity of these attacks is variable and related to a multitude of exacerbating factors and triggers, such as dental and surgical manipulation, stress or trauma, menses, medications, and infections. Attacks can be precipitated by estrogen in particular, either through endogenous increases during menses or pregnancy or via exogenous sources, such as oral contraceptives or hormone replacement therapy.[29]

It is estimated that up to 50% of HAE attacks may be precipitated by trauma or stress, although others may be spontaneous in nature.[30] Symptom onset typically begins in early life, with up to 75% of patients experiencing their first attack before the age of 15.[14]

HAE-1 constitutes approximately 80% to 85% of all cases of HAE. The swelling may present early in life, often by the teen years, and can increase after puberty. Like other causes of angioedema, episodes may be precipitated by physical or emotional stressors. HAE-2 represents 15% to 20% of all HAE cases and is similar in presentation to HAE-1. Angioedema may present in the face, extremities, abdomen, and other organ systems, with the concern of laryngeal edema and asphyxiation, as in the case of HAE-1.

The most common presentation is that of nonemergent angioedema resulting in impairment in quality of life with discomfort, immobility, and disfigurement, and the inability to attend work or school.[31]

Abdominal attacks occurring in up to 93% of patients with HAE[29] can present with mild to severe spasmodic pain and may be associated with gastrointestinal upset and even intestinal obstruction; hypovolemic shock may result from the extravasation of fluids.[30] These attacks can often be confused with appendicitis or cholecystitis, resulting in unnecessary surgical interventions,[18,20] and even psychiatric referrals.[4]

Laryngeal attacks with respiratory impairment and the risk of asphyxiation is the most feared complication of these attacks, because these patients may require intubation and even tracheotomies.[30] It is estimated that up to 50% of HAE patients will experience at least 1 laryngeal episode within their lifetime.[25]

In distinguishing between angioedema with impaired C1INH (ie, HAE-1 and HAE-2) versus HAE-nC1NH, there are several clinical characteristics that allow for differentiation: In the case of angioedema with normal C1INH, patients are usually women, presenting in adulthood. These individuals will more frequently present with facial swelling, specifically of the tongue, with the risk of asphyxiation and laryngeal involvement. In cases of HAE-nC1NH, there tends to be less abdominal involvement, and no antecedent erythema marginatum.[32] Furthermore, the presentation and penetrance of the disease have been noted to be quite low, because patients have presented in later decades of life, with normal or low levels of estrogen.[4,33,34]

Acquired agioedema Acquired forms of C1INH-deficiency, a bradykinin-mediated angioedema, typically present later in life in individuals with no family history of hereditary angioedema. It has been associated with lymphoproliferative and hematologic diseases. The estimated prevalence is reported to be 1:500,000,[14] although it is thought to be underrecognized. Although the clinical presentation is similar to HAE, these individuals may present with additional symptoms of their underlying malignancy. Reduced antigenic and functional levels of C1-INH with low C4 complement levels (with a normal C3), in addition to having low levels of C1q, help distinguish acquired forms of angioedema from hereditary angioedema.[14] Supporting evidence for acquired forms may be obtained from complete blood counts with lymphocyte immunophenotyping, blood films, inflammatory markers, antinuclear antibodies and complement levels, rheumatoid factor, and serum protein electrophoresis with immunofixation studies, as addressed in the consideration of diagnostic measures in the evaluation of idiopathic and acquired causes of angioedema. Consideration may also be given to bone marrow biopsies and targeted imaging studies to evaluate for underlying malignancies and lymphoproliferative disorders, such as lymphoma, multiple myeloma, and monoclonal gammopathy of uncertain significance, as a cause of acquired forms.[5,12,35,36] Hereditary and acquired forms of C1 esterase inhibitor

(C1-INH) deficiency maybe difficult to distinguish clinically, although laboratory parameters and a family history of HAE aid in the differentiation between subtypes.

Angiotensin-converting enzyme–inhibitor induced angioedema It is estimated that 0.1% to 0.7% of patients on ACE inhibitors (and less commonly angiotensin receptor blockers) may develop angioedema,[37] typically occurring within the first week to month of treatment,[3] although some cases may develop after years of therapy. Typical areas of involvement occur in the face, lips, and tongue with the risk of fatalities due to laryngeal involvement; in comparison to other angioedema subtypes, there is relative sparing of the gut and genital mucosa.[5] Several risk factors have been identified, including prior head and neck surgery,[38] external trauma,[38] increasing age, and female gender, and even smoking.[39–43] There is a preponderance among African Americans[3,14] thought to be secondary to polymorphisms found in the aminopeptidase P gene, which plays an essential role in the metabolism of ACE inhibitors.[3] There is no strong evidence to suggest that there may be a dose-dependent relationship nor has it been shown to occur with greater frequency with specific ACE inhibitors or with the timing of medications.[44]

DIAGNOSTIC EVALUATION OF BRADYKININ-MEDIATED ANGIOEDEMA

To distinguish between hereditary angioedema subtypes, laboratory investigation begins with a screening measurement of a serum C4 complement level as well as obtaining diagnostic antigenic and functional levels of the inhibitor of the first component of the complement pathway, C1-INH. To note, as the sensitivity of a low C4 level in diagnosing HAE is estimated at approximately 86%,[45] pursuing further investigations with chromogenic assays to confirm diagnosis is recommended.

Both HAE-1 and HAE-2 are associated with decreased levels of C4 at baseline and during acute episodes; however, although HAE-1 is characterized by a low antigenic level of C1-INH, HAE-2 often has normal or even elevated antigenic levels of C1-INH with a functional impairment.[3] HAE-nC1INH differs in that it maintains normal C4 complement levels with unaffected C1-INH antigenic and functional levels (**Table 3**).[46]

In acquired forms of angioedema, the evaluation of complement levels, specifically C3, C4, and C1q, are useful markers because these are often reduced.[3] In ACE-inhibitor induced and idiopathic bradykinin-mediated angioedema, the diagnosis is reliant on the clinical history because laboratory parameters, including serum complements, C1-INH antigenic and functional levels, serum tryptase, and urine histamine will all be normal.[3]

In cases of where angioedema is thought to be bradykinin mediated but investigations are normal and family history is negative, an empiric trial of treatment directed toward bradykinin-mediated angioedema could be considered.

Table 3
Laboratory findings in hereditary angioedema

	C4	C1-INH Antigen	C1INH Function
HAE-1	↓	↓	↓
HAE-2	↓	Normal or ↑	↓
HAE-nC1INH			
FXII mutation	Normal	Normal	Normal
Unknown cause	Normal	Normal	Normal

From Betschel S, Badiou J, Binkley K, et al. Canadian hereditary angioedema guideline. Allergy Asthma Clin Immunol 2014;10(1):50; with permission.

Essential Components of the Clinical History

An accurate diagnosis is reliant on obtaining the clinical history of angioedema with or without urticaria, time to onset, and the response to treatment with antihistamines, corticosteroids, and epinephrine. A diagnosis of hereditary or acquired angioedema must be considered if allergic causes and histaminergic mechanisms are unlikely.

Pertinent information in the history includes the following[5]:

1. Characterization of the angioedema
   - Association with/without urticaria
   - Age of onset
   - Time to onset
   - Sites affected (head and neck, peripheries, gastrointestinal tract)
   - Associated symptoms suggestive of an alternative cause or underlying malignancy
2. Response to corticosteroids, antihistamines, and epinephrine
3. Potential triggers or exacerbating factors:
   - Medications (NSAIDs, ACE inhibitors, angiotensin II receptor blockers, narcotics, estrogen-containing oral contraceptives, antibiotics, neuromuscular blocking agents, latex)[4]
   - Dental or surgical manipulation (as they are often triggers of HAE)
   - Stress (mental or physical)
   - Exercise
   - Infections
   - Menses
   - Alcohol
   - Past history of IgE-mediated reactions to foods, medications, insect stings, latex
4. Comorbidities (including autoimmunity and malignancies)

A detailed family history is also essential because HAE-1 and II are of autosomal dominant inheritance; however, up to 25% of all cases may result from spontaneous mutations.[34]

An Algorithmic Approach to Diagnosis of Angioedema

In encountering a patient with angioedema, one should first establish its association with or without urticaria; if the patient presents with urticaria, histaminergic causes should be explored. Once this differentiation has been made and angioedema mimickers ruled out, this allows for the further classification of angioedema without wheals. If angioedema is unresponsive to antihistamines, corticosteroids, and epinephrine, bradykinin-mediated angioedema should be considered. It is through the appreciation of angioedema subtypes, their respective pathophysiologies, and differentiating features that allows us to apply an algorithmic approach to obtain an accurate diagnosis (**Fig. 5**).[47–49] Given the potential severity and life-threatening nature of angioedema, it is essential for medical professionals to reach a prompt diagnosis and initiate the appropriate course of action.

FUTURE CONSIDERATIONS

The accurate diagnosis of angioedema is reliant on a thorough patient and family history, allowing for further stratification through response to treatment, laboratory parameters, and investigations (**Table 4**).[18,50–52] Angioedema has been shown to significantly impair one's quality of life,[53] affecting both their physical and their mental well-being, and thus establishing a prompt diagnosis, and a treatment plan is

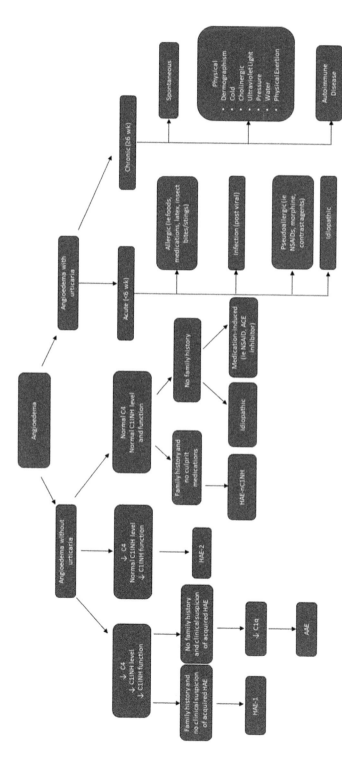

Fig. 5. Angioedema algorithm. AAE, acquired angioedema; C1INH, C1 esterase inhibitor; HAE-nC1NH, hereditary angioedema with normal C1 esterase inhibitor.

Table 4
Summary of the laboratory profiles and evaluation of angioedema

Type	Clinical Description	Antigenetic C1-INH	Functional C1-INH	C1q level	C3	C4	Other Markers
Histamine-mediated							
Allergic angioedema (with urticaria)	• Typically accompanied by urticaria (which may be vasculitic) • Possibly pruritic • May be associated with anaphylaxis • 24–72-h duration • Responsive to antihistamines or corticosteroids	NL	NL	NL	NL‡	NL‡	Urine histamine and serum tryptase often elevated ‡Complements may be low in hypocomplementemic urticarial vasculitis
Bradykinin-mediated							
Acquired	• Appears in middle age or later • No family history • Unresponsive to antihistamines or corticosteroids • May be associated with an underlying malignancy or autoimmune disorders	Low/NL	Low	Low	Low/NL	Low	A malignancy workup should be considered
ACE inhibitor-induced	• Typically occurs within the first 3 mo of ACE-inhibitor initiation • No urticaria • More common in blacks and smokers • Commonly involves the lips, tongue, face	NL	NL	NL	NL	NL	
HAE-1	• Recurrent episodes of swelling of any body part • Attacks preceded by erythema marginatum in up to ½ of cases • No urticaria • Attacks may last as long as 3–5 d • Symptoms begin in childhood and worsen in puberty • Positive family history • AD inheritance (although up to 25% can occur de novo) • Unresponsive to antihistamines or corticosteroids	Low	Low	NL	NL	Low	

	Notes						
HAE-2	• Same as T1	NL	Low	NL	NL	Low	
HAE-nC1INH	• Same as T1, but may have estrogen sensitivity • Positive family history • Associated with mutations in Factor II • Recurrent tongue swelling is a cardinal symptom • Unresponsive to antihistamines or corticosteroids	NL	NL	NL	NL	NL	
Not conclusively mediated by histamine or bradykinin							
Idiopathic	• ≥3 episodes of swelling/y • No apparent cause • Urticaria present in up to 50% • Responsive to antihistamines or corticosteroids	NL	NL	NL	NL	NL	
Pseudo allergic	• Urticaria is typically present • Mechanism is thought to be due to an increase of cysteinyl-leukotrienes (eg, NSAID-induced angioedema)	NL	NL	NL	NL	NL	
Gleich syndrome	• Episodic swelling with eosinophilia and elevated IgM	NL	NL	NL	NL	NL	Elevated IgM antibody, with eosinophilia

Abbreviation: AD, autosomal dominant.

essential. Targeted therapies are under development in the management of both hereditary and acquired forms for the prevention and management of attacks, with the hopes of improving the lives of affected individuals. Research endeavors related to angioedema are aimed at gaining a comprehensive understanding of the pathophysiology and perhaps genetic contributions underlying this disease process to better assist in its evaluation, diagnosis, and management. The establishment of an angioedema registry would aid in the better understanding of the clinical presentation, importance of quality-of-life measures, as well as responses to treatments. It is through a commitment to basic sciences research, clinical trials, and an appreciation for the disease burden that advancements in this field will continue to gain momentum.

REFERENCES

1. Donati M. De medica historia mirabile. Mantua Osana.1586;VII: Cap iii:304.
2. Osler W. Hereditary angioneurotic edema. Am J Med Sci 1888;95:362.
3. Bernstein JA, Moellman J. Emerging concepts in the diagnosis and treatment of patients with undifferentiated angioedema. J Emerg Med 2012;5:39.
4. Gompels MM, Lock RJ, Abinun M, et al. C1 inhibitor deficiency: consensus document. Clin Exp Immunol 2005;139(3):379–94.
5. Grigoriadou S, Longhurst HJ. Clinical immunology review series: an approach to the patient with angio-oedema. Clin Exp Immunol 2008;155(3):367–77.
6. Abbas AK, Pober JS, Lichtman AH. Cellular and molecular immunology. Philadelphia: Saunders/Elsevier; 2010.
7. Morgan BP. Hereditary angioedema—therapies old and new. N Engl J Med 2010; 363(6):581–3.
8. Asero R, Riboldi P, Tedeschi A, et al. Chronic urticaria: a disease at a crossroad between autoimmunity and coagulation. Autoimmun Rev 2007;7:71–6.
9. von Bubnoff D, Novak N, Kraft S, et al. The central role of FcepsilonRI in allergy. Clin Exp Dermatol 2003;28(2):184–7.
10. Deadock SJ. An approach to the patient with urticaria. Clin Exp Immunol 2008; 153(2):151–61.
11. Bas M, Adams V, Suvorava T, et al. Nonallergic angioedema: role of bradykinin. Allergy 2007;62(8):842–56.
12. Cicardi M, Zingale L, Zanichelli A, et al. C1 inhibitor: molecular and clinical aspects. Springer Semin Immunopathol 2005;27(3):286–98.
13. Zuraw BL. Hereditary angioedema. N Engl J Med 2008;359(10):1027–36.
14. Hoyer C, Hill MR, Kaminski ER. Angio-oedema: an overview of differential diagnosis and clinical management. Contin Educ Anaesth Crit Care Pain 2012; 12(6):307–11.
15. Gompels MM, Lockr RJ, Morgan JE, et al. A multicentre study of the diagnostic efficiency of serological investigations for C1 inhibitor deficiency. J Clin Pathol 2002;55:145–7.
16. Tarzi MD, Hickey A, Forster T, et al. An evaluation of tests used for the diagnosis and monitoring of C1 inhibitor deficiency: normal serum C4 does not exclude hereditary angio-oedema. Clin Exp Immunol 2007;149(3):513–6.
17. Bork K, Witzke G. Shortened activated partial thromboplastin time may help in diagnosing hereditary and acquired angioedema. Int Arch Allergy Immunol 2016;170:101–7.
18. Nzeako U. Diagnosis and management of angioedema with abdominal involvement: a gastroenterology perspective. World J Gastroenterol 2010;16(39): 4913–21.

19. Venzor J, Lee WL, Huston DP. Urticarial vasculitis. Clin Rev Allergy Immunol 2002; 23(2):201–16.
20. Nzeako UC, Frigas E, Tremaine WJ. Hereditary angioedema as a cause of transient abdominal pain. J Clin Gastroenterol 2002;34:57–61.
21. Kaplan AP, Greaves MW. Angioedema. J Am Acad Dermatol 2005;53:373–88 [quiz: 389-92].
22. Kowalski ML, Asero R, Bavbek S, et al. Classification and practical approach to the diagnosis and management of hypersensitivity to nonsteroidal anti-inflammatory drugs. Allergy 2013;68(10):1219–32.
23. Moore-Robinson M, Warin RP. Effect of salicylates in urticaria. Br Med J 1967;4: 262–4.
24. Zingale LC, Beltrami L, Zanichelli A, et al. Angioedema without urticaria: a large clinical survey. CMAJ 2006;175(9):1065–70.
25. Agostoni A, Aygoren-Pursun E, Binkley KE, et al. Hereditary and acquired angioedema: problems and progress: proceedings of the third C1 esterase inhibitor deficiency workshop and beyond. J Allergy Clin Immunol 2004;114(3 Suppl): S51–131.
26. Banerji A, Sheffer AL. The spectrum of chronic angioedema. Allergy Asthma Proc 2009;30(1):11–6.
27. Wakisaka M, Shuto M, Abe H, et al. Computed tomography of the gastrointestinal manifestation of hereditary angioedema. Radiat Med 2008;26(10):618–21.
28. Hereditary Angioedema. USHAEA.org website. Available at: http://www.haea. org. Accessed December 11, 2016.
29. Bork K, Meng G, Staubach P, et al. Hereditary angioedema: new findings concerning symptoms, affected organs, and course. Am J Med 2006;119(3):267–74.
30. Frank MM, Gelfand JA, Atkinson JP. Hereditary angioedema: the clinical syndrome and its management. Ann Intern Med 1976;84(5):580–93.
31. Castaldo AJ, Vernon MK, Lumry WR, et al. Humanistic burden of hereditary angioedema [abstract]. Ann Allergy Asthma Immunol 2009;102:A92 [abstract: P249].
32. Weldon D. Differential diagnosis of angioedema. Immunol Allergy Clin North Am 2006;26(4):603–13.
33. Miranda AR, de Ue APF, Sabbag DV, et al. Hereditary angioedema type III (estrogen-dependent) report of three cases and literature review. An Bras Dermatol 2013;88(4):578–84.
34. Bork K. Diagnosis and treatment of hereditary angioedema with normal C1 inhibitor. All Asth Clin Immunol 2010;6:5.
35. Cicardi M, Aberer W, Banerji A, et al. Classification, diagnosis, and approach to treatment for angioedema: consensus report from the Hereditary Angioedema International Working Group. Allergy 2014;69(5):602–16.
36. Cicardi M, Banerji A, Bracho F, et al. Icatibant, a new bradykinin-receptor antagonist, in hereditary angioedema. N Engl J Med 2010;363:532–41.
37. Byrd JB, Adam A, Brown NJ. Angiotensin-converting enzyme inhibitor–associated angioedema. Immunol Allergy Clin North Am 2006;264:725–37.
38. Megerain CA, Arnold JE, Berger M. Angioedema: 5 years' experience, with a review of the disorder's presentation and treatment. Laryngoscope 1992;102: 256–60.
39. Kostis JB, Packer M, Black HR, et al. Omapatrilat and enalapril in patients with hypertension: the omapatrilat cardiovascular treatment vs. enalapril (OCTAVE) trial. Am J Hypertens 2004;17:103–11.

40. Brown NJ, Ray WA, Snowden M, et al. Black Americans have an increased rate of angiotensin converting enzyme inhibitor-associated angioedema. Clin Pharmacol Ther 1996;60:8–13.

41. Gibbs CR, Lip GY, Beevers DG. Angioedema due to ACE inhibitors: increased risk in patients of African origin. Br J Clin Pharmacol 1999;48:861–5.

42. Lefebvre J, Murphey LJ, Hartert TV, et al. Dipeptidyl peptidase IV activity in patients with ACE-inhibitor-associated angioedema. Hypertension 2002;39:460–4.

43. Morimoto T, Gandhi TK, Fiskio JM, et al. An evaluation of risk factors for adverse drug events associated with angiotensin-converting enzyme inhibitors. J Eval Clin Pract 2004;10:499–509.

44. Macaulay TE, Dunn SP. Cross-reactivity of ACE inhibitor–induced angioedema with ARBs. US Pharmacist; 2007. Available at: https://www.uspharmacist.com/article/cross-reactivity-of-ace-inhibitorinduced-angioedema-with-arbs. Accessed November 10, 2016.

45. Li H, Busse P, Lumry W, et al. Comparison of chromogenic and ELISA functional C1 inhibitor tests in diagnosis hereditary angioedema. J Allergy Clin Immunol Pract 2015;3(2):200–5.

46. Betschel S, Badiou J, Binkley K, et al. Canadian HAE Guidelines. Allergy Asthma Clin Immunol 2014;10(1):50.

47. Zuraw BL, Bernstein JA, Lang DM, et al, American Academy of Allergy, Asthma and Immunology. A focused parameter update: hereditary angioedema, acquired c1 inhibitor deficiency, and angiotensin-converting enzyme inhibitor-associated angioedema. J Allergy Clin Immunol 2013;131(6):1491–3.

48. Fu L, Freedman-Kalchman T, Betschel S, et al. Review of hereditary angioedema. Lymphosign J 2016;3(2):47–53.

49. Rasmussen ER, Bindslev-Jenson C, Bygum A. Angioedema – assessment and treatment. Tidsskr Nor Laegeforen 2012;132:2391–5.

50. Weis M. Clinical review of hereditary angioedema: diagnosis and management. Postgrad Med 2009;121(6):113–20.

51. Johnston D. Diagnosis and management of hereditary angioedema. J Am Osteopath Assoc 2011;111:28–36.

52. Nzeako UC, Frigas E, Tremaine WJ. Hereditary angioedema: a broad review for clinicians. Arch Intern Med 2001;161(20):2417–29.

53. Lumry WR, Miller DP, Newcomer S, et al. Quality of life in patients with hereditary angioedema receiving therapy for prevention of attacks. Allergy Asthma Proc 2014;35(5):371–6.

Histaminergic Angioedema

Paula J. Busse, MD*, Tukisa Smith, MD

KEYWORDS

- Angioedema • Histamine • Urticaria • Histaminergic • Inducible urticaria
- Spontaneous urticaria

KEY POINTS

- Angioedema, which involves the development of nonpitting edema affecting deep cutaneous layers and mucosal tissues, can be histamine or bradykinin mediated. Determining the subtype of angioedema is critical for the choice of therapy.
- Histamine-mediated angioedema is clinically distinguished by symptoms' duration (acute and chronic), the presence or absence of urticaria, and whether there are known factors inducing symptoms or not.
- Histaminergic angioedema is secondary to mast-cell and basophil activation, and therefore, the mainstay of treatment includes antihistamines, corticosteroids, and epinephrine (for emergency use).

INTRODUCTION

Angioedema is a result of increased vascular permeability with subsequent extravasation of intravascular fluid into the surrounding tissues, which include the skin, gastrointestinal (GI) tract, and upper airways.[1] Angioedema can be broadly classified into 3 categories based on the underlying mechanism and mediator producing symptoms:

1. Histaminergic angioedema
2. Bradykinin-mediated angioedema (eg, hereditary angioedema [HAE], ACE inhibitor–induced angioedema, and acquired C1 inhibitor deficiency, discussed in other articles in this issue)
3. Causes of unknown mechanisms.

There are certain key features of symptom onset and presentation that help evaluate whether angioedema is histamine or bradykinin mediated (**Table 1**). Determining

Disclosure Statement: P.J. Busse has received consulting fees from Shire and CSL Behring; research funding from Shire and CSL Behring.
Division of Allergy and Clinical Immunology, Icahn School of Medicine at Mount Sinai, 1425 Madison Avenue, New York, NY 10029-6574, USA
* Corresponding author.
E-mail address: paula.busse@mssm.edu

Immunol Allergy Clin N Am 37 (2017) 467–481
http://dx.doi.org/10.1016/j.iac.2017.03.001
0889-8561/17/© 2017 Elsevier Inc. All rights reserved.

immunology.theclinics.com

Table 1
Differential features of histamine- versus bradykinin-mediated angioedema

Features	Histamine Mediated	Bradykinin Mediated
Rash	Urticaria	No urticaria, occasional erythema marginatum
Family history	Atopy	Recurrent angioedema in 75% of patients with HAE
Onset/duration of symptoms	Rapid; 24–48 h	Typically slower; 3–5 d
Pruritus	Present	None, may be painful
Response to antihistamines/CS/Epi	+	−

Abbreviations: CS, corticosteroids; Epi, epinephrine.

the category of angioedema is critical for its treatment. For example, histaminergic angioedema responds to antihistamines, corticosteroids, or epinephrine, whereas bradykinin-mediated angioedema requires medications targeting this peptide and/or its pathway. Histaminergic angioedema is the most common form of angioedema and is subdivided into acute and chronic forms based on its duration of symptoms (acute <6 weeks; chronic >6 weeks) (**Fig. 1**). Histaminergic angioedema is further classified as that occurring with or without urticaria (wheals). The organization of histaminergic angioedema in this review is derived from several sources: the 2014 Hereditary Angioedema International Working (HAWK) Group consensus report on angioedema,[2] the European Academy of Allergy and Clinical Immunology (EAACI), Global Allergy and Asthma European Network (GA²LEN), European Dermatology Forum (EDF), World Allergy Organization (WAO) urticaria guideline (EAACI/GA²LEN/EDF/WAO),[3] and the American Academy of Allergy, Asthma, and Immunology/American College of Allergy, Asthma, and Immunology Joint Task Force (JTF) guideline.[4] This article reviews the

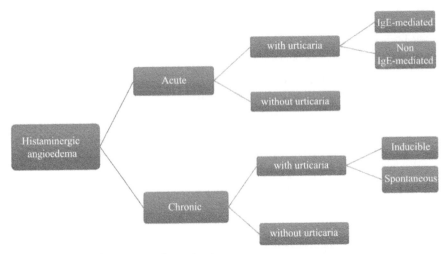

Fig. 1. Schematic of histaminergic angioedema.

subtypes of histaminergic angioedema, its presentation, pathophysiology, evaluation, and management.

ACUTE ANGIOEDEMA
Allergic (Immunoglobulin E–Mediated) Angioedema

Presentation
Allergic angioedema is frequently accompanied by urticaria; isolated angioedema as a result of an allergic response is relatively uncommon. As a mast-cell–mediated process with release of mediators, including histamine, leukotrienes, heparin, platelet-activating factor, and cytokines, there are often other symptoms, including flushing, generalized pruritus, and bronchospasm. GI pain and vomiting may be present when allergens are ingested. Often, allergic urticaria is self-limited, with symptoms resolving within 24 hours. Allergic angioedema may persist beyond this time period, but unlike bradykinin-mediated angioedema that can last 3 to 5 days, the former does not typically last longer than 24 to 48 hours. Symptoms will reoccur upon repeated exposure to the allergen or to cross-reacting allergens.[5] The allergic reaction can progress to anaphylaxis (defined by specific criteria[6,7]), which may result in death without appropriate treatment. Urticaria is characterized by an erythematous raised rash with an initial pale center (wheal) with intense itching. Urticarial wheals that do not have a "fleeting" nature (ie, the site of the hive on the skin does not return to its normal appearance <24 hours), those that are nonblanching, or those that leave pigment changes should prompt suspicion of an alternative diagnosis. Angioedema does not characteristically itch and is more likely to be painful. Patients typically experience angioedema and urticarial symptoms within 30 to 60 minutes after allergen exposure. Specific foods (eg, peanuts, tree nuts, shellfish, fish in adults, and milk, egg, soy in children), insect venom, medications (eg, penicillins), and environmental allergens, are common triggers producing immediate symptoms. However, some patients may develop a delayed allergic reaction, occurring 2 to 6 hours after ingestion of certain meats (eg, lamb, beef, pork) if they have developed a hypersensitivity to the carbohydrate galactose-alpha 1,3-galactose.[8]

Pathophysiology
Allergic angioedema is secondary to production of antigen (Ag)-specific immunoglobulin E (IgE) molecules in predisposed individuals following an initial exposure to this Ag. After secretion by B-lymphocytes, most Ag-specific IgE bind to their high-affinity FcεR1 receptors on the surface of mast cells and basophils, whereas the remainder circulates in the serum. When the patient is reexposed to the Ag, bound IgE molecules recognize specific proteins on the Ag, binding them, and bringing the IgE molecules closer together on the cell surface, a term called "cross-linking." Cross-linking activates intracellular tyrosine kinases and protein kinase C, increasing intracellular calcium. This cascade degranulates mast cells and basophils with subsequent release of histamine, tryptase, and chymase, which comprise the "early phase" of the reaction and begins transcription of specific cytokines (eg, interleukin [IL]-1, -2, -5, -6, -8, -9, -13), chemokines, and growth factors (eg, vascular endothelial growth factor) that initiate the "late-phase" reaction.[9] Histamine binds to selective H1-receptors, inducing vasodilation and increasing blood flow and vascular permeability of the submucosal or subcutaneous capillaries, and/or postcapillary venules. Vessel leakage is dependent on the integrity of the endothelial cell-cell junction and cell-surface expression of the transmembrane adhesive protein, vascular endothelial (VE) cadherin. Histamine also phosphorylates VE-cadherin, which weakens this tight barrier.[10,11] In addition, histamine stimulates nitric oxide expression, increasing blood

flow.[12] The net result is increased plasma extravagation to nearby tissues, producing angioedema. The underlying mechanism of IgE-dependent angioedema and urticaria is the same; the former occurs in deeper levels of the dermis and subcutaneous tissues, whereas the latter occurs in the superficial papillary and middermis layers. Pruritus is the result of histamine-stimulated afferent type-C fibers and the release of substance P.

There are multiple downstream effects of mast cell and basophil activation. For example, several cell types, including neutrophils, eosinophils, macrophages, basophils, and CD4+ T cells, form a nonnecrotizing infiltration into local tissue.[13] This pathology differs from urticarial vasculitis in which there is vessel wall necrosis.[14,15] Activation of neutrophils may further increase vascular leak through release of leukotriene B4.[16]

Nonallergic Mast-Cell–Mediated Acute Angioedema

Presentation

Acute urticaria and angioedema occur less frequently from direct mast cell activation or a non-IgE-mediated process. These triggers include some medications and infections, but more frequently, the cause remains unidentified. Depending on the inciting event, some reactions can occur within 1 hour after exposure to the precipitant, for example, drugs (eg, opiates, vancomycin, nonsteroidal anti-inflammatory drugs [NSAIDs] [see Cosby Stone and Nancy J. Brown's article, "ACE-Inhibitor and Other Drug-Associated Angioedema," in this issue"]), or radiocontrast dye. Bacterial, viral, parasitic, or fungal pathogens such as *Helicobacter pylori*, Streptococci, Staphylococci, *Giardia lamblia*, *Mycoplasma pneumoniae*, hepatitis virus, Norovirus, Parvovirus B19, Anisakis simplex, and *Entamoeba* ssp have been implicated as underlying causes, but are not routinely screened for as a cause.[3] Respiratory tract infections are most commonly reported in children with symptoms of acute urticaria and angioedema, but may also be a trigger in adults.[17–19]

Pathophysiology

Although mast cells are typically activated by cross-linking of their FcεRI and IgE-Ag complexes, there are alternative pathways. Anaphylatoxins C3a and C5a, the human antibacterial peptide B-defensin, and substance P degranulate mast cells.[20–22] In addition, murine studies have demonstrated that influenza A–specific IgG2$_a$, IgG2$_b$, and IgG$_1$ induced mast cell degranulation.[23] After mast cell activation, the subsequent inflammatory cascades are similar to IgE-triggered events.

CHRONIC ANGIOEDEMA
Histamine-Mediated Angioedema with Chronic Urticaria

Angioedema is present in approximately 40% to 50% of patients with chronic urticaria (CU).[24,25] The following section focuses on the classifications of CU, based on 2 guidelines: the EAACI/GA^{2}LEN/EDF/WAO[3] and the JFT,[4] which share many similarities, but differ on some recommendations. Persistent symptoms greater than 6 weeks is a widely agreed upon definition of CU. However, the frequency of symptoms per week is not listed in either guideline, but most reports suggest that it should be present for at least 3 days per week.[26–29] Both guidelines divide CU into 2 subtypes, but differ slightly in the terminology. The EAACI/GA^{2}LEN/EDF/WAO groups CU into "inducible" urticaria (CIU), in which symptoms are secondary to specific triggers (ie, UV light, cold, exercise, pressure, water, vibration), and "spontaneous" urticaria (CSU), which develops without identifiable provocation[3] (**Table 2**). The JFT uses the terminology "continuous" and "intermittent."[4]

Table 2
Classification of chronic urticaria with angioedema

Types	Subtypes	Eliciting Factors
Spontaneous	Chronic spontaneous urticaria	No identifiable trigger
Inducible		
Physical urticarias	Cold contact urticaria	Exposure of skin to cold air, cold objects, or cold liquids
	Delayed pressure urticaria	Vertical pressure and wheal development 30 min to 12 h after exposure
	Heat contact urticaria	Direct skin contact with a warm object
	Solar urticaria	Exposure of skin to sunlight of specific wavelength
	Symptomatic dermatographic urticaria	Mechanical stroking or scratching of the skin surface and wheal development 1–5 min after exposure
	Vibratory urticaria	Exposure to mechanical vibration
Other inducible urticarias	Aquagenic urticaria	Skin contact with water at any temperature
	Cholinergic urticaria	Elevation of body temperature with exercise, hot water, strong emotion, or spicy food
	Exercise-induced anaphylaxis/ urticaria	Exertional activity

Physical Urticaria

Presentation

The physical urticarias are a heterogeneous subgroup in which wheals are reproducibly induced by specific physical stimuli, such as mechanical pressure (ie, rubbing, vibration), thermal stimuli (ie, cold, heat), or sunlight.[30,31] Approximately 25% of patients with CU demonstrate symptoms consistent with physical urticaria, most frequently in young adults.[31] Physical urticaria may be present in children, but it occurs less frequently than in adults.[32]

The severity of physical urticaria varies and may depend on the subtype, and in some cases, may be potentially life threatening (ie, airway swelling after a cold exposure in patients with cold induced urticaria). Angioedema is usually limited to the stimulus site; however, generalized symptoms can occur. Dermographism is the most common form of physical urticaria, which presents with raised urticarial wheals on the site of the skin after scratching or stroking (termed "simple dermographism") or extensive wheals in areas extending beyond those which were stimulated (termed "symptomatic dermographism").[33] Triggers of dermographism include itching dry skin, resulting in linear urticarial lesions, and rubbing of clothing, or direct pressure upon the skin (for example, sitting on a chair). Delayed-pressure urticaria/angioedema, occasionally classified as a subtype of symptomatic dermographism, is an erythematous swelling of the skin developing approximately 4 to 6 hours after application of pressure. Its causes are similar to those producing dermographism, including sitting for prolonged periods of time, tight clothing, or carrying heavy bags. Vibratory angioedema is the development of pruritus with subsequent angioedema (usually without urticaria) after exposure to a vibratory stimulus.[34,35] Triggers include mowing the lawn, bicycle riding, or jack-hammering. Other less common causes of physical urticaria include local heat, in which there is direct contact of the skin with a warm stimulus, and aquagenic urticaria, secondary to contact with water of any temperature, with symptoms developing ~20 to 30 minutes after exposure.

Pathophysiology
The underlying pathophysiologies of the physical urticaria/angioedema are not completely understood, but likely involve mast-cell stimulation with release of its vasoactive mediators, much like nonallergic acute angioedema/urticaria. Mast cell involvement is suggested by increased serum histamine in patients with dermographism or aquagenic urticaria.[36–40] In addition, increased IL-1 and IL-17 expression[41,42] and activation of blood coagulation and fibrinolysis (demonstrated by increased platelet activation and increased D-dimer)[43,44] contribute to the underlying pathogenesis of delayed pressure urticaria/angioedema.

Cholinergic Urticaria

Presentation
Cholinergic urticaria is characterized by numerous small (1-3 mm) punctuate wheals surrounded by large flares. Lesions typically originate in the trunk. Cholinergic urticaria is often associated with increased body temperature secondary to hot water, exercise, and sometimes strong emotions and spicy foods. Cholinergic urticaria can present with cholinergic urticaria with angioedema, but this does not occur commonly. However, recently a group of patients developing cholinergic urticaria with angioedema, most commonly around the eyelids, and some with anaphylaxis, after exercise or bathing in hot water were identified.[45]

Pathophysiology
Acetylcholine (Ach) stimulation is thought to be an underlying cause of cholinergic urticaria, as demonstrated by patients developing local urticaria after Ach injection.[46] Some patients appear to have an IgE-mediated reaction to their sweat,[47] whereas others appear to have a non-IgE-mediated mechanism through modification of their Ach receptor, especially in those with concomitant hypohidrosis.[48]

Chronic Spontaneous Urticaria with Angioedema

Presentation/pathophysiology
The presentation of CSU is similar to that of CIU, except that there is no identifiable trigger. Similar to CIU, a lowered mast cell activation threshold is central to the underlying pathophysiology of CSU. However, the exact trigger of mast cell degranulation in CSU is not clear. In approximately one-third of patients, there are IgG autoantibodies targeted to either IgE or the α subunit of the high-affinity IgE receptor (FcεRIα), which then activates mast cells and basophils.[49,50] Although IgE sensitization does not play a role in the pathogenesis of CSU, skin biopsies of patients have demonstrated an eosinophilic and T helper 2 cellular infiltrate. This may be due to activation of the innate pathway, through release of IL-25, IL-33, and thymic stromal lymphopoietin by stromal cells, including endothelial and epithelial cells.[51] In vitro studies have also suggested activation of the classical complement pathway.[52,53] In some patients, there is evidence of systemic inflammation as demonstrated by increased plasma IL-6, which may correlate with disease activity.[54,55]

It is postulated that a proportion of CSU patients might have underlying emotional stress as an exacerbating factor, but it is unlikely to be the sole cause of disease.[16,56,57] Previous studies have reported that half of patients with CSU experience high rates of anxiety, depression, and somatoform disorders.[58,59] However, it is important to note that CU also induces emotional stress and produces a substantial negative impact on the quality of life for patients.[60] Therefore, there is likely an important bidirectional relationship between urticaria and emotional stress.

Histamine-Mediated Angioedema Without Urticaria

Presentation

A focus of the 2014 HAWK conference was to classify angioedema without wheals.[2] At this meeting, the term *idiopathic histaminergic acquired angioedema (IH-AAE)* was developed to describe patients who develop recurrent episodes of angioedema without urticaria, whose symptoms are controlled by antihistamines and in whom there is no identifiable cause such as allergy or physical stimuli.[2] The prevalence of IH-AAE is not well established, possibly due to its recent terminology. However, in a large referral center for angioedema, 379 of the 1058 consecutively referred patients for angioedema without urticaria over a 10-year period had chronic angioedema without cause that responded to antihistamine therapy, thus fulfilling the definition of IH-AAE.[61] This group of patients typically present with angioedema developing rapidly, reaching its maximum swelling by 6 hours, and resolving within 24 hours. The face is the most commonly affected body site, but it may involve the extremities and GI mucosa (in <30% of patients). Although it may be present in patients of all ages, it is typically detected in those between 36 and 42 years of age.[62] In children, histaminergic angioedema without urticaria can occur, but is less common than in adults.[63]

DIAGNOSIS AND EVALUATION

Acute Angioedema

A directed patient history is critical to determine whether angioedema may be histamine or bradykinin mediated (see **Table 1**). Patients should be asked if they have ingested foods before symptoms onset, with particular attention to those more commonly allergenic (eg, peanut, tree nuts, fish, shellfish in adults, and milk and egg in children). An IgE-mediated reaction typically occurs within 1 hour after ingestion and can be later assessed by skin prick testing or serum evaluation for food Ag-specific IgE. Medication history should address recent use of antibiotics, NSAIDs, or ACE-I. Not all medication-related angioedema or urticaria episodes are IgE mediated. Commonly, IgE-mediated reactions to antibiotics are from penicillins, for which IgE evaluation has been established.[64] Many other medication reactions producing angioedema/urticaria are not IgE mediated, such as NSAIDs; therefore, skin prick testing or serum evaluate is not helpful. ACE-I–induced angioedema is bradykinin mediated. Routine blood work (ie, complete blood cell counts, complete metabolic panels) testing in acute urticaria is not indicated.[3] The occurrence of urticaria with angioedema favors a histamine-mediated process. However, the nature of the urticarial lesions should be assessed for their duration and response to antihistamines in order to exclude other causes, such as urticarial vasculitis, as mentioned previously. In addition, the patient's response to antihistamines, corticosteroids, or epinephrine is an important clue to suggest a histamine-driven disorder, whereas a lack of response suggests a bradykinin-mediated process.

Chronic Angioedema

The underlying cause of chronic histamine-mediated angioedema is rarely determined. As a result, extensive laboratory testing is not recommended by the EAACI/GA²LEN/EDF/WAO and JTF guidelines.[3,4] Both recommend a complete blood cell count with differential, complete metabolic panel, and erythrocyte sedimention rate or C-reactive protein (to exclude the possibility of an underlying chronic condition that could be treated). The JTF guideline also recommends a thyroid-stimulating hormone test and liver function enzymes test. Although many patients with CSU may have an underlying autoimmune component, its evaluation is not recommended because it does not change the choice of therapy. Antibodies that are commonly detected include antithyroid antibodies and IgG autoantibodies against the high-affinity IgE receptor (FcεR1) or IgE; the presence of the latter autoantibodies often results in a positive autologous serum skin test (ASST).[65] The incidence in an autoimmune component in children is not well established. However, a single-site retrospective study of 100 children (ages 0.7 months to 17 years), evaluated for CSU over a 7-year period, noted that 46.7% had a positive ASST.[66]

The natural history of CU is difficult to predict, and the duration of symptoms varies. Some patients may have a 30% to 50% remission rate within 3 years after symptom onset,[67,68] whereas others remain symptomatic 10 years beyond their initial presentation.[69] However, there are several factors that can aid in prediction of prognosis. Patients who experience urticaria with angioedema appear to suffer symptoms longer than those with urticaria alone,[70] or those with angioedema alone.[57,68] Patients with milder disease, compared with those with moderate to severe symptoms, tend to have a shorter symptom duration.[70,71] Furthermore, patients with a component of autoreactivity (ie, positive ASST or antibodies against FcεR1 or IgE) tend to have a longer duration of disease than those without.[72,73] Finally, the presence of physical urticaria with other forms of angioedema/urticaria often prolongs duration of disease.[68,71,74]

Differential Diagnosis

Besides distinguishing histaminergic angioedema from bradykinin-mediated angioedema, which can be suggested by urticaria in the former, and a lack of response to antihistamines and corticosteroids in the latter, there are other disorders that can present with urticarial-like lesions and angioedema. Examples include mastocytosis (which can present with pigmented papules), urticarial vasculitis, and systemic lupus erythematosus. Cryoglobulinemia may cause cold-induced urticarial or vasculitic lesions in patients with hepatitis B or C. Gleich syndrome is episodic angioedema with eosinophilia. Hypereosinophilic syndrome is a group of disorders due to increased production of eosinophils with tissue deposition, resulting in a variety of symptoms depending on the subtype, which can include recurrent urticaria and angioedema. The Muckle-Wells syndrome is rare, but involves mutations in cryopyrin, and patients may have periodic urticarial eruptions and persistent swelling (potentially due to amyloid deposition). Patients also experience sensorineural hearing loss and arthritis. In addition, angioedema must be distinguished from edema, either protein-losing conditions or cardiac failure. Unlike angioedema, edema is pitting, typically symmetric (ie, both extremities), and in dependent areas of the body. Obstructive abnormalities such as superior vena cava syndrome or head and neck tumors may present with persistent swelling.

MANAGEMENT
Acute Management

An acute episode of angioedema/urticaria can occur as the initial episode or as a flare of chronic disease. If patients require an emergency room visit for their symptoms, the evaluation must first address their airway for potential asphyxiation due to airway edema. Evaluation includes monitoring physical symptoms which may suggest airway compromise such as change in voice, difficulty swallowing, or stridor.[75] If there are signs of significant airway compromise, intubation should be considered. Next, the patient's vital signs should be accessed for hypotension and tachycardia, which occur due to profound vasodilation and increased vascular permeability, producing fluid shifts. After the patient's airway and hemodynamic status are evaluated and stabilized, the history and physical examination should distinguish between histamine- and bradykinin-mediated angioedema (see **Table 1**), which will guide subsequent management. Unfortunately, at the present time, there are no blood tests to provide rapid results to help determine the underlying mediator (eg, histamine vs bradykinin); therefore, the history is critical. In addition, measurement of histamine and bradykinin in the serum is difficult to perform and not commercially available. However, certain laboratory work can be performed, such as serum tryptase (elevated in mast-cell activation) and C4 (decreased in HAE type I and II, and acquired C1-INH deficiency; see Iris M. Otani and Aleena Banerji's article, "Acquired C1 Inhibitor Deficiency"; and Kaplan AP and Joseph K's article, "Pathogenesis of Hereditary Angioedema: The Role of the Bradykinin Forming Cascade," in this issue), which can be followed up on upon discharge. Performing serum Ag–specific IgE testing during an acute episode does not provide rapid results either and should be done approximately 2 or more weeks after the episode for most reliable results. If the patient has been previously evaluated for angioedema/urticaria, it is more likely that the underlying mediator producing symptoms has been established.

The following section briefly discusses additional measures in acute management of angioedema/urticaria. However, the reader is referred to recently published summary statements on the management of angioedema in an emergency room for a detailed discussion on the approach and treatment of patients with acute angioedema in this setting.[75,76] The treatment of histamine-mediated acute angioedema and urticaria is directed by its symptoms. For patients presenting with airway compromise and/or a systemic reaction (ie, hypotension, tachycardia, GI symptoms), intramuscular epinephrine is required and can be repeated every 5 to 15 minutes as needed.[75] Antihistamines are also administered during an acute histamine-mediated episode of angioedema/urticaria of any severity. Only first-generation antihistamines (ie, diphenhydramine) are available for intravenous administration, but second-generation antihistamines, only available in oral preparations, are equally effective. Glucocorticoids are often administered to prevent late-phase reactions that can occur 4 to 6 hours after the initial response. In cases in which patients have required epinephrine, they must be prescribed and taught how to use a self-injectable epinephrine before discharge. Patients should also be referred to an allergist upon discharge who can follow up for evaluation of IgE sensitizations and continued management. If the allergic trigger is identified during the emergency visit, the patient must be educated to avoid it upon discharge.

Chronic Management

The preventive management of histaminergic angioedema is extrapolated from the management of CU. The first-line therapy is second-generation, nonsedating antihistamines. There are no preferred antihistamines, and all theoretically should work equally well; therefore, the drug selection must be based on a discussion between the patient and physician. Some patients report an improved response to certain antihistamines, or tolerate specific preparations, or there may be a cost issue. The initial daily dose to administer antihistamine may be at the standard dose, or in some patients, higher based on their severity of symptoms (ie, twice a day). At the initial treatment, any triggers of symptoms should be avoided. However, it is not necessary to recommend that patients avoid all potential triggers of angioedema/urticaria if they have not experienced symptoms with their exposure (eg, asking all patients with urticaria to avoid NSAIDs if they have previously tolerated them). If patients have persistent symptoms after a 2-week daily preventative antihistamine treatment, the next step is to titrate the dosage up to a maximum of 4-fold the standard labeled dose.[32] The JFT guidelines also recommend the addition of H2-blockers, first-generation antihistamines before bed, and leukotriene-modifying agents if 4 times a day dosing is not completely effective.[4,77] However, first-generation antihistamines present the risk of increased sedation, which is particularly problematic for older patients.[3] A short course of oral corticosteroids may be considered in these patients; topical corticosteroids are typically of little benefit. If symptoms persist despite these measures, the addition of omalizumab (Xolair, Genentech, Inc, San Francisco, CA, USA), an anti-IgE antibody, can be considered. Omalizumab has strong data suggesting its efficacy in CU and is approved by the US Food and Drug Administration and the European Medicines Agency for the treatment of adults and adolescents who have refractory CIU and CSU.[78] Case reports suggest that it improves physical urticarias, including solar, cold, delayed pressure, dermographism, and cholinergic urticaria as well as idiopathic histaminergic angioedema.[79–81] Importantly, it has also been demonstrated to significantly improve quality of life of patients with urticaria.[82] In addition to omalizumab, cyclosporine A (CsA) should be considered. Before the availability and approval of omalizumab, CsA was often used with improvement of symptoms. However, CsA is an immunosuppressant and is frequently associated with adverse effects, including GI disturbances, elevated blood pressure, and possible nephrotoxicity, limiting its use. Additional anti-inflammatory and other immunosuppressants, such as dapsone, sulfasalazine, hydroxychloroquine, colchicine, anti-tumor necrosis factor-α, and the anti-CD20 biologic, rituximab, have shown improvement in smaller, less rigorous studies of patients with CU and are therefore not frequently prescribed.[4,83,84] If the treatment with high-dose antihistamines and alternative agents does not improve symptoms, an alternative diagnosis should be considered, including evaluation for a bradykinin-mediated process.

The optimal duration of therapy for chronic histamine-mediated angioedema/urticaria is unknown. Providers should consider tapering therapy once patients have achieved complete symptom control to assess for disease remission. Fortunately, there are few adverse effects with long-term second-generation antihistamine use. Omalizumab can be reduced in frequency of interval injections from every 4 weeks to every 6 weeks or longer with continued monitoring for symptom recurrence.[77]

SUMMARY

Histaminergic angioedema is the most common form of angioedema and must be distinguished from bradykinin-mediated forms for optimal treatment. Histaminergic angioedema is frequently associated with urticaria. It is classified upon its duration of symptoms into either acute or chronic. Evaluation for an IgE-mediated process is indicated in the evaluation of acute angioedema/urticaria. Chronic angioedema/urticaria may be classified as inducible or spontaneous forms, based on its trigger or lack of known trigger, and can occur in the presence or absence of urticaria. Unfortunately, the underlying trigger of CU is frequently not able to be determined, and bothersome symptoms may persist for several months to years. Consequently, this disorder has a significant negative impact on patients' quality of lives. The mainstay of treatment of histaminergic angioedema/urticaria is second-generation antihistamines to prevent symptoms (chronic cases) as well as for treatment of acute attacks. All patients with previous episodes of airway angioedema from a histamine-mediated process must be prescribed and taught how to self-inject epinephrine and be educated on its indications for use.

REFERENCES

1. Kaplan AP, Greaves MW. Angioedema. J Am Acad Dermatol 2005;53(3):373–88 [quiz: 389–92].
2. Cicardi M, Aberer W, Banerji A, et al. Classification, diagnosis, and approach to treatment for angioedema: consensus report from the Hereditary Angioedema International Working Group. Allergy 2014;69(5):602–16.
3. Zuberbier T, Aberer W, Asero R, et al. The EAACI/GA(2) LEN/EDF/WAO Guideline for the definition, classification, diagnosis, and management of urticaria: the 2013 revision and update. Allergy 2014;69(7):868–87.
4. Bernstein JA, Lang DM, Khan DA, et al. The diagnosis and management of acute and chronic urticaria: 2014 update. J Allergy Clin Immunol 2014;133(5):1270–7.
5. Kaplan AP. Angioedema. World Allergy Organ J 2008;1(6):103–13.
6. Sampson HA, Muñoz-Furlong A, Bock SA, et al. Symposium on the definition and management of anaphylaxis: summary report. J Allergy Clin Immunol 2005; 115(3):584–91.
7. Sampson HA, Muñoz-Furlong A, Campbell RL, et al. Second symposium on the definition and management of anaphylaxis: summary report–Second National Institute of Allergy and Infectious Disease/Food Allergy and Anaphylaxis Network symposium. J Allergy Clin Immunol 2006;117(2):391–7.
8. Commins SP, Satinover SM, Hosen J, et al. Delayed anaphylaxis, angioedema, or urticaria after consumption of red meat in patients with IgE antibodies specific for galactose-alpha-1,3-galactose. J Allergy Clin Immunol 2009;123(2):426–33.
9. Sismanopoulos N, Delivanis DA, Alysandratos KD, et al. Mast cells in allergic and inflammatory diseases. Curr Pharm Des 2012;18(16):2261–77.
10. Ashina K, Tsubosaka Y, Nakamura T, et al. Histamine induces vascular hyperpermeability by increasing blood flow and endothelial barrier disruption in vivo. PLoS One 2015;10(7):e0132367.
11. Orsenigo F, Giampietro C, Ferrari A, et al. Phosphorylation of VE-cadherin is modulated by haemodynamic forces and contributes to the regulation of vascular permeability in vivo. Nat Commun 2012;3:1208.
12. Durán WN, Breslin JW, Sánchez FA. The NO cascade, eNOS location, and microvascular permeability. Cardiovasc Res 2010;87(2):254–61.
13. Kaplan A. Inflammation in chronic urticaria is not limited to the consequences of mast cell (or basophil) degranulation. Clin Exp Allergy 2010;40(6):834–5.
14. Haas N, Schadendorf D, Henz BM. Differential endothelial adhesion molecule expression in early and late whealing reactions. Int Arch Allergy Immunol 1998; 115(3):210–4.
15. Ito Y, Satoh T, Takayama K, et al. Basophil recruitment and activation in inflammatory skin diseases. Allergy 2011;66(8):1107–13.
16. Powell RJ, Leech SC, Till S, et al. BSACI guideline for the management of chronic urticaria and angioedema. Clin Exp Allergy 2015;45(3):547–65.
17. Aoki T, Kojima M, Horiko T. Acute urticaria: history and natural course of 50 cases. J Dermatol 1994;21(2):73–7.
18. Ricci G, Giannetti A, Belotti T, et al. Allergy is not the main trigger of urticaria in children referred to the emergency room. J Eur Acad Dermatol Venereol 2010; 24(11):1347–8.
19. Sakurai M, Oba M, Matsumoto K, et al. Acute infectious urticaria: clinical and laboratory analysis in nineteen patients. J Dermatol 2000;27(2):87–93.

20. Chen X, Niyonsaba F, Ushio H, et al. Antimicrobial peptides human beta-defensin (hBD)-3 and hBD-4 activate mast cells and increase skin vascular permeability. Eur J Immunol 2007;37(2):434–44.

21. Hartmann K, Henz BM, Krüger-Krasagakes S, et al. C3a and C5a stimulate chemotaxis of human mast cells. Blood 1997;89(8):2863–70.

22. Matsuda H, Kawakita K, Kiso Y, et al. Substance P induces granulocyte infiltration through degranulation of mast cells. J Immunol 1989;142(3):927–31.

23. Grunewald SM, Hahn C, Wohlleben G, et al. Infection with influenza a virus leads to flu antigen-induced cutaneous anaphylaxis in mice. J Invest Dermatol 2002; 118(4):645–51.

24. Fine LM, Bernstein JA. Urticaria guidelines: consensus and controversies in the European and American Guidelines. Curr Allergy Asthma Rep 2015;15(6):30.

25. Maurer M, Church MK, Marsland AM, et al. Questions and answers in chronic urticaria: where do we stand and where do we go? J Eur Acad Dermatol Venereol 2016;30(Suppl 5):7–15.

26. Chansakulporn S, Pongpreuksa S, Sangacharoenkit P, et al. The natural history of chronic urticaria in childhood: a prospective study. J Am Acad Dermatol 2014; 71(4):663–8.

27. Confino-Cohen R, Chodick G, Shalev V, et al. Chronic urticaria and autoimmunity: associations found in a large population study. J Allergy Clin Immunol 2012; 129(5):1307–13.

28. Kaplan AP. Chronic urticaria: pathogenesis and treatment. J Allergy Clin Immunol 2004;114(3):465–74 [quiz: 475].

29. Powell RJ, Du Toit GL, Siddique N, et al. BSACI guidelines for the management of chronic urticaria and angio-oedema. Clin Exp Allergy 2007;37(5):631–50.

30. Abajian M, Młynek A, Maurer M. Physical urticaria. Curr Allergy Asthma Rep 2012;12(4):281–7.

31. Abajian M, Schoepke N, Altrichter S, et al. Physical urticarias and cholinergic urticaria. Immunol Allergy Clin North Am 2014;34(1):73–88.

32. Khakoo G, Sofianou-Katsoulis A, Perkin MR, et al. Clinical features and natural history of physical urticaria in children. Pediatr Allergy Immunol 2008;19(4): 363–6.

33. Schoepke N, Młynek A, Weller K, et al. Symptomatic dermographism: an inadequately described disease. J Eur Acad Dermatol Venereol 2015;29(4):708–12.

34. Dice JP. Physical urticaria. Immunol Allergy Clin North Am 2004;24(2):225–46, vi.

35. Patterson R, Mellies CJ, Blankenship ML, et al. Vibratory angioedema: a hereditary type of physical hypersensitivity. J Allergy Clin Immunol 1972;50(3):174–82.

36. Botto NC, Warshaw EM. Solar urticaria. J Am Acad Dermatol 2008;59(6):909–20 [quiz: 921–2].

37. Garafalo J, Kaplan AP. Histamine release and therapy of severe dermatographism. J Allergy Clin Immunol 1981;68(2):103–5.

38. Hawk JL, Eady RA, Challoner AV, et al. Elevated blood histamine levels and mast cell degranulation in solar urticaria. Br J Clin Pharmacol 1980;9(2):183–6.

39. Metzger WJ, Kaplan AP, Beaven MA, et al. Hereditary vibratory angioedema: confirmation of histamine release in a type of physical hypersensitivity. J Allergy Clin Immunol 1976;57(6):605–8.

40. Shelley WB, Rawnsley HM. Aquagenic urticaria. Contact sensitivity reaction to water. JAMA 1964;189:895–8.

41. de Koning HD, van Vlijmen-Willems IM, Rodijk-Olthuis D, et al. Mast-cell interleukin-1β, neutrophil interleukin-17 and epidermal antimicrobial proteins in the

neutrophilic urticarial dermatosis in Schnitzler's syndrome. Br J Dermatol 2015; 173(2):448–56.

42. Lenormand C, Lipsker D. Efficiency of interleukin-1 blockade in refractory delayed-pressure urticaria. Ann Intern Med 2012;157(8):599–600.

43. Kasperska-Zajac A, Brzoza Z, Rogala B. Increased concentration of platelet-derived chemokines in serum of patients with delayed pressure urticaria. Eur Cytokine Netw 2008;19(2):89–91.

44. Kasperska-Zając A, Jasinska T. Analysis of plasma D-dimer concentration in patients with delayed pressure urticaria. J Eur Acad Dermatol Venereol 2011;25(2): 232–4.

45. Washio K, Fukunaga A, Onodera M, et al. Clinical characteristics in cholinergic urticaria with palpebral angioedema: report of 15 cases. J Dermatol Sci 2016; 85:135–7.

46. Bito T, Sawada Y, Tokura Y. Pathogenesis of cholinergic urticaria in relation to sweating. Allergol Int 2012;61(4):539–44.

47. Fukunaga A, Bito T, Tsuru K, et al. Responsiveness to autologous sweat and serum in cholinergic urticaria classifies its clinical subtypes. J Allergy Clin Immunol 2005;116(2):397–402.

48. Itakura E, Urabe K, Yasumoto S, et al. Cholinergic urticaria associated with acquired generalized hypohidrosis: report of a case and review of the literature. Br J Dermatol 2000;143(5):1064–6.

49. Kaplan AP, Greaves M. Pathogenesis of chronic urticaria. Clin Exp Allergy 2009; 39(6):777–87.

50. Hide M, Francis DM, Grattan CE, et al. Autoantibodies against the high-affinity IgE receptor as a cause of histamine release in chronic urticaria. N Engl J Med 1993;328(22):1599–604.

51. Kay AB, Clark P, Maurer M, et al. Elevations in T-helper-2-initiating cytokines (interleukin-33, interleukin-25 and thymic stromal lymphopoietin) in lesional skin from chronic spontaneous ('idiopathic') urticaria. Br J Dermatol 2015;172(5): 1294–302.

52. Asero R, Tedeschi A, Lorini M, et al. Chronic urticaria: novel clinical and serological aspects. Clin Exp Allergy 2001;31(7):1105–10.

53. Ferrer M, Nakazawa K, Kaplan AP. Complement dependence of histamine release in chronic urticaria. J Allergy Clin Immunol 1999;104(1):169–72.

54. Kasperska-Zajac A, Sztylc J, Machura E, et al. Plasma IL-6 concentration correlates with clinical disease activity and serum C-reactive protein concentration in chronic urticaria patients. Clin Exp Allergy 2011;41(10):1386–91.

55. Daschner A, Rodero M, De Frutos C, et al. Different serum cytokine levels in chronic vs. acute Anisakis simplex sensitization-associated urticaria. Parasite Immunol 2011;33(6):357–62.

56. Ozkan M, Oflaz SB, Kocaman N, et al. Psychiatric morbidity and quality of life in patients with chronic idiopathic urticaria. Ann Allergy Asthma Immunol 2007; 99(1):29–33.

57. Maurer M, Weller K, Bindslev-Jensen C, et al. Unmet clinical needs in chronic spontaneous urticaria. A GA(2)LEN task force report. Allergy 2011;66(3):317–30.

58. Picardi A, Abeni D. Stressful life events and skin diseases: disentangling evidence from myth. Psychother Psychosom 2001;70(3):118–36.

59. Staubach P, Dechene M, Metz M, et al. High prevalence of mental disorders and emotional distress in patients with chronic spontaneous urticaria. Acta Derm Venereol 2011;91(5):557–61.

60. Baiardini I, Pasquali M, Braido F, et al. A new tool to evaluate the impact of chronic urticaria on quality of life: chronic urticaria quality of life questionnaire (CU-QoL). Allergy 2005;60(8):1073–8.

61. Mansi M, Zanichelli A, Coerezza A, et al. Presentation, diagnosis and treatment of angioedema without wheals: a retrospective analysis of a cohort of 1058 patients. J Intern Med 2015;277(5):585–93.

62. Cicardi M, Bergamaschini L, Zingale LC, et al. Idiopathic nonhistaminergic angioedema. Am J Med 1999;106(6):650–4.

63. Ertoy Karagol HI, Yilmaz O, Bakirtas A, et al. Angioedema without urticaria in childhood. Pediatr Allergy Immunol 2013;24(7):685–90.

64. Macy E. Penicillin allergy: optimizing diagnostic protocols, public health implications, and future research needs. Curr Opin Allergy Clin Immunol 2015;15(4):308–13.

65. Konstantinou GN, Asero R, Maurer M, et al. EAACI/GA(2)LEN task force consensus report: the autologous serum skin test in urticaria. Allergy 2009;64(9):1256–68.

66. Sahiner UM, Civelek E, Tuncer A, et al. Chronic urticaria: etiology and natural course in children. Int Arch Allergy Immunol 2011;156(2):224–30.

67. Quaranta JH, Rohr AS, Rachelefsky GS, et al. The natural history and response to therapy of chronic urticaria and angioedema. Ann Allergy 1989;62(5):421–4.

68. Kozel MM, Mekkes JR, Bossuyt PM, et al. Natural course of physical and chronic urticaria and angioedema in 220 patients. J Am Acad Dermatol 2001;45(3):387–91.

69. Humphreys F, Hunter JA. The characteristics of urticaria in 390 patients. Br J Dermatol 1998;138(4):635–8.

70. Toubi E, Kessel A, Avshovich N, et al. Clinical and laboratory parameters in predicting chronic urticaria duration: a prospective study of 139 patients. Allergy 2004;59(8):869–73.

71. van der Valk PG, Moret G, Kiemeney LA. The natural history of chronic urticaria and angioedema in patients visiting a tertiary referral centre. Br J Dermatol 2002;146(1):110–3.

72. Kulthanan K, Jiamton S, Thumpimukvatana N, et al. Chronic idiopathic urticaria: prevalence and clinical course. J Dermatol 2007;34(5):294–301.

73. Sabroe RA, Seed PT, Francis DM, et al. Chronic idiopathic urticaria: comparison of the clinical features of patients with and without anti-FcepsilonRI or anti-IgE autoantibodies. J Am Acad Dermatol 1999;40(3):443–50.

74. Amin P, Levin L, Holmes SJ, et al. Investigation of patient-specific characteristics associated with treatment outcomes for chronic urticaria. J Allergy Clin Immunol Pract 2015;3(3):400–7.

75. Moellman JJ, Bernstein JA, Lindsell C, et al. A consensus parameter for the evaluation and management of angioedema in the emergency department. Acad Emerg Med 2014;21(4):469–84.

76. Pedrosa M, Prieto-García A, Sala-Cunill A, Spanish Group for the Study of Bradykinin-Mediated Angioedema (SGBA) and the Spanish Committee of Cutaneous Allergy (CCA). Management of angioedema without urticaria in the emergency department. Ann Med 2014;46(8):607–18.

77. Khan DA. Alternative agents in refractory chronic urticaria: evidence and considerations on their selection and use. J Allergy Clin Immunol Pract 2013;1(5):433–40.e1.

78. Beck LA, Bernstein JA, Maurer M. A review of international recommendations for the diagnosis and management of chronic urticaria. Acta Derm Venereol 2016; 97(2):149–58.

79. Vestergaard C, Toubi E, Maurer M, et al. Treatment of chronic spontaneous urticaria with an inadequate response to H1-antihistamines: an expert opinion. Eur J Dermatol 2016;27(1):10–9.

80. von Websky A, Reich K, Steinkraus V, et al. Complete remission of severe chronic recurrent angioedema of unknown cause with omalizumab. J Dtsch Dermatol Ges 2013;11(7):677–8.

81. Sands MF, Blume JW, Schwartz SA. Successful treatment of 3 patients with recurrent idiopathic angioedema with omalizumab. J Allergy Clin Immunol 2007; 120(4):979–81.

82. Maurer M, Sofen H, Ortiz B, et al. Positive impact of omalizumab on angioedema and quality of life in patients with refractory chronic idiopathic/spontaneous urticaria: analyses according to the presence or absence of angioedema. J Eur Acad Dermatol Venereol 2016. [Epub ahead of print].

83. Ghazan-Shahi S, Ellis AK. Severe steroid-dependent idiopathic angioedema with response to rituximab. Ann Allergy Asthma Immunol 2011;107(4):374–6.

84. Mallipeddi R, Grattan CE. Lack of response of severe steroid-dependent chronic urticaria to rituximab. Clin Exp Dermatol 2007;32(3):333–4.

Angiotensin-converting Enzyme Inhibitor and Other Drug-associated Angioedema

Cosby Stone Jr, MD, MPH[a], Nancy J. Brown, MD[b],*

KEYWORDS

- Angioedema • ACE inhibitor • Bradykinin • NSAID • Leukotriene • Drug
- Medication

KEY POINTS

- Drug-induced angioedema should be characterized as being either allergic (histamine mediated) or nonallergic mechanism based, because this guides therapeutic decision making.
- Nonsteroidal antiinflammatory drugs can cause angioedema in a susceptible host via shifts in the synthesis of prostaglandins and leukotrienes.
- A growing number of drugs cause angioedema by inhibiting pathways involved in the degradation of bradykinin and substance P.
- B_2 receptor antagonism and kallikrein inhibition have not been as successful in the treatment of drug-induced bradykinin-mediated angioedema as in hereditary angioedema.

INTRODUCTION

Angioedema is characterized by localized deep dermal, subcutaneous, and/or mucosal edema resulting from increased vasodilatation and vascular permeability. Nonsteroidal antiinflammatory drugs (NSAIDs), β-lactam antibiotics, non–β lactam antibiotics, and angiotensin-converting enzyme (ACE) inhibitors are the most common classes of drugs that cause angioedema.[1–3] Drug-induced angioedema is best categorized as allergic or nonallergic. The most common form of allergic angioedema is caused by immunoglobulin (Ig)-E–mediated degranulation of mast cells and release of histamine (type I hypersensitivity) in response to a drug and this is the most common

Disclosure: The authors have nothing to disclose.
[a] Division of Allergy, Pulmonary and Critical Care Medicine, Vanderbilt University Medical Center, 1161 21st Avenue South T-1218, Medical Center North, Nashville, TN 37232-2650, USA;
[b] Department of Medicine, Vanderbilt University Medical Center, 1161 21st Avenue South D-3100, Medical Center North, Nashville, TN 37232, USA
* Corresponding author.
E-mail address: nancy.j.brown@vanderbilt.edu

Immunol Allergy Clin N Am 37 (2017) 483–495
http://dx.doi.org/10.1016/j.iac.2017.04.006
0889-8561/17/© 2017 Elsevier Inc. All rights reserved.

cause of angioedema caused by β-lactam and other antibiotics.[1] Nonallergic forms of angioedema result as a consequence of the underlying mechanism of the drug. NSAIDs may cause hypersensitivity reactions but angioedema results more commonly because of the diversion of arachidonic acid metabolism from the cyclooxygenase (COX) pathway to the leukotriene pathway. ACE inhibitor–associated angioedema results from decreased degradation of kinins and other vasoactive peptides; there is a growing list of drugs that affect these pathways.

Clinically it is important to distinguish between allergic and nonallergic forms of drug-induced angioedema because the response to therapy differs dramatically. Allergic forms of drug-induced angioedema respond to antihistamines, glucocorticosteroids, and epinephrine, whereas nonallergic forms do not. The presence of pruritus or urticaria in a patient without a prior history of urticaria suggests an allergic form of drug-induced angioedema. For completeness, **Table 1** provides a list of drugs that cause histamine-mediated angioedema (see Busse PJ, Smith T: Histaminergic Angioedema, in this issue). This article focuses primarily on nonallergic forms of drug-induced angioedema.

ANGIOEDEMA ASSOCIATED WITH NONSTEROIDAL ANTIINFLAMMATORY DRUG USE

The European Academy of Allergy and Clinical Immunology Task Force on NSAID Hypersensitivity proposed classifying immediate-type NSAID reactions into 5 categories, 3 of which can present with angioedema.[4]

Table 1
Drugs that cause histamine-medicated angioedema and their reported mechanisms of mast cell degranulation

IgE Mediated	Direct Mast Cell Degranulation, Via G-Protein–coupled Receptors or Other Means	Drug Causes Histamine-mediated Angioedema Only Rarely, or Mechanism is Not Understood
Antimicrobials: Penicillins,[51] cephalosporins,[52] Carbapenems,[51] fluoroquinolones,[53] sulfonamides,[54] vancomycin,[55] macrolides[56] Chemotherapeutics: Platinum-based agents,[57] paclitaxel,[58] cetuximab (via galactose-alpha-1, 3-galactose allergy)[59] Procedural medications: Radiographic contrast,[60] opiates,[61] neuromuscular blocking agents,[62] NSAIDs[63] Gastrointestinal medications: Proton pump inhibitors,[64] polyethylene glycol[65]	Antimicrobials: Fluoroquinolones,[66] sulfonamides[67] (especially in patients with human immunodeficiency virus), vancomycin[a] (associated with worsening of angioedema only)[3,55] Chemotherapeutics: Paclitaxel[a,68] Procedural medications: Radiographic contrast,[a,69] opiates,[a,70] neuromuscular blocking agents[a,66]	Antimicrobials: Daptomycin,[71] clindamycin,[72] chloramphenicol[73] Antituberculosis agents: Rifampicin,[74] streptomycin,[75] ethambutol,[76] isoniazid[77] Immune suppressants: Tacrolimus,[78] sirolimus[79] Psychiatric medications: selective serotonin reuptake inhibitors[80] Procedural medications: Hyaluronidase[81]

[a] For medications with more than 1 reported mechanism, what seems to be the most common mechanism for reactions is indicated when that information is available.

The most straightforward category is single NSAID–induced urticaria/angioedema or anaphylaxis in a patient with no underlying urticaria/angioedema disease. The patient presents with angioedema while using a particular NSAID, or NSAIDs that are structurally related, and has no symptoms when using NSAIDs of different structural categories. The mechanism for these structure-specific reactions is generally thought to be IgE-mediated type I hypersensitivity, and IgEs specific for pyrazolone NSAIDs have been detected in patients who developed angioedema or urticaria while taking these agents.[5] Identification of IgEs specific for other families of NSAIDs has not been reported. Treatment involves the discontinuation and avoidance of NSAIDs structurally related to the NSAID that caused symptoms.

The second category is NSAID-induced urticaria/angioedema (NIUA). These reactions occur in patients without an underlying tendency to chronic urticaria/angioedema in response to the ingestion of structurally dissimilar NSAIDs. The mechanism underlying this class effect is thought to involve an imbalance in arachidonic acid metabolism or altered leukotriene/prostaglandin binding to receptors. Angioedema results when COX-1 inhibition shunts arachidonic acid away from the production of antiinflammatory prostaglandin D_2 and E_2 and toward increases in production of leukotriene B_4, C_4, and D_4, which cause vasodilation, plasma leakage, and angioedema. Genetic variants in the genes encoding *ALOX5*, *ALOX15*, *PTGDR*, *PTGER1*, and *CYSLTR1* have been reported to predispose patients to this condition.[6–8] Typically, acetaminophen is safe for use in this group of patients, and selective COX-2 inhibitors have also been used safely.

The third category of NSAID-induced angioedema occurs in patients with underlying chronic urticaria and/or angioedema, and is called NSAID-exacerbated cutaneous disease. The mechanism seems to be similar to NIUA, whereby alterations in the balance between prostaglandin and leukotriene production leads to angioedema in patients with an underlying predisposition to angioedema or urticaria. For this reason, NSAID desensitization is not effective in this type of patient.[9] Treatment should emphasize control of underlying chronic angioedema/urticaria.

ANGIOTENSIN-CONVERTING ENZYME INHIBITOR–ASSOCIATED ANGIOEDEMA
Clinical Features of Angiotensin-converting Enzyme Inhibitor–associated Angioedema

ACE inhibitor–associated angioedema typically involves the lips, tongue, or face. Angioedema may also involve the bowel; in this case, the patient may present with abdominal pain and symptoms of obstruction and the diagnosis can be made by identification of bowel edema on computed tomography scan with resolution of symptoms after discontinuation of the ACE inhibitor. The risk of ACE inhibitor–associated angioedema is greatest during the first week to month of exposure, but angioedema can occur at any time,[10–12] suggesting that an additional inciting factor may contribute to the pathogenesis of ACE inhibitor–associated angioedema (discussed later). Angioedema may remit spontaneously, but, if ACE inhibitor use is continued, angioedema typically recurs.[11] Many patients with ACE inhibitor–associated angioedema do not present for acute care. However, among those presenting for emergency treatment, up to 16% require intubation and 1% require tracheostomy.[13] Rapid evolution of symptoms; involvement of the tongue, soft palate or larynx; and symptoms of drooling or respiratory distress are associated with a higher risk of intubation.[13]

Epidemiology of and Risk Factors for Angiotensin-converting Enzyme Inhibitor–associated Angioedema

The reported incidence of ACE inhibitor–associated angioedema ranges from 0.1% to 0.7% in retrospective studies to as high as 2.8% to 6% in prospective clinical trials.[14–17] The incidence of ACE inhibitor–associated angioedema is 4.5-fold to 5-fold higher in patients of African descent compared with white people.[12,18–20] ACE inhibitor–associated angioedema is uncommon in Asian patients. A history of seasonal allergies, antihistamine use, or corticosteroid use is associated with an increased risk of ACE inhibitor–associated angioedema.[10,20] At least 1 group has reported that there is seasonal variation in presentation of ACE inhibitor–associated angioedema, with increased presentations occurring during months with high pollen counts, especially in patients with allergic sensitization.[21] Smokers and former smokers are at increased risk of ACE inhibitor–associated angioedema, whereas patients with type 2 diabetes mellitus are at decreased risk.[10,12,20] Immunosuppressant use, rheumatoid arthritis, and history of transplant have been associated with an increased risk of ACE inhibitor–associated angioedema.[10,22,23]

Pathophysiology of Angiotensin-converting Enzyme Inhibitor–associated Angioedema

Like hereditary angioedema, ACE inhibitor–associated angioedema is thought to result from excess bradykinin. Hereditary angioedema results from increased production of kinins[24]; however, ACE inhibitor–associated angioedema results from decreased degradation of bradykinin and other vasoactive ACE substrates, such as substance P (**Fig. 1**). Bradykinin increases vascular permeability through its B_2 receptor and via sensitization of the transient potential vanilloid receptor I (TRPV1).[25]

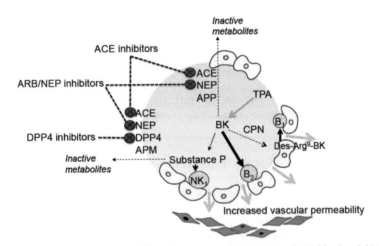

Fig. 1. Hypothesized mechanism of drug-induced angioedema mediated by bradykinin and substance P. Activation of kallikrein-kinin system results in the generation of bradykinin (BK). TPA can also increase BK through formation of plasmin and the contact system. BK activates the B_2 and transient potential vanilloid receptor I (TRPV1; not shown) receptors to cause vasodilation and vascular permeability, and stimulates the release of substance P. Substance P increases vascular permeability via the neurokinin 1 (NK_1) receptor. BK is inactivated primarily by ACE, aminopeptidase P (APP), and neutral endopeptidase (NEP), whereas substance P is inactivated by ACE, NEP, and dipeptidyl peptidase 4 (DPP4). Inhibition of these enzymes by drugs in a susceptible patient can lead to accumulation of BK and/or substance P and angioedema. Des-Arg⁹-BK, a metabolite of BK by carboxypeptidase N (CPN), may also cause angioedema via the B_1 receptor. ARB, angiotensin receptor blocker; APM, aminopeptidase M; TPA, tissue plasminogen activator. (*Modified from* Brown NJ. Angiotensin-converting enzyme inhibitor-associated angioedema. Immunol Allergy Clin North Am 2010;30(Suppl 1):46; with permission.)

Bradykinin also stimulates the release of substance P from nerve terminals; substance P increases vascular permeability by activating the NK_1 receptor.[26,27] Treatment with a bradykinin B_2 receptor antagonist, a TRPV1 antagonist, or a substance P NK_1 receptor antagonist decreases ACE inhibitor–associated angioedema in rodent models.[25–28]

ACE degrades both bradykinin and substance P. When ACE is inhibited, other enzymes, such as neprilysin (neutral endopeptidase [NEP]), carboxypeptidase N, and aminopeptidase P (APP), degrade and inactivate bradykinin. Likewise, during ACE inhibition, dipeptidyl peptidase 4 (DPP4) and NEP inactivate substance P. Genetic or environmental factors that decrease the activity of these non-ACE enzyme pathways in the degradation of bradykinin and substance P would be expected to increase the risk of angioedema.

Genetics of Angiotensin-converting Enzyme Inhibitor–associated Angioedema

Sturrock and colleagues[29] reported that a 9-base-pair deletion variant in the bradykinin B_2 receptor, leading to increased transcription and increased sensitivity to bradykinin, is associated with ACE inhibitor–associated angioedema in black and mixed-race South Africans.[30] The investigators did not find an association between an ACE insertion/deletion polymorphism and ACE inhibitor–associated angioedema, but reported that ACE activity was significantly decreased in patients with angioedema compared with ACE inhibitor–treated controls without angioedema.[30] Other groups have not observed an association between variants in the genes encoding ACE or the bradykinin B_2 receptor and ACE inhibitor–associated angioedema.[31,32]

Several candidate gene studies have examined the association between functional variants in genes encoding enzymes involved in the degradation of bradykinin and other vasoactive peptides and ACE inhibitor–associated angioedema. Duan and colleagues[33] identified a single nucleotide polymorphism (SNP) in the gene encoding membrane APP (XPNPEP2, -2399C > A, or rs3788853), which is associated with decreased plasma APP activity and angioedema in families associated with anaphylactoid reactions during hemodialysis and/or angioedema during ACE inhibitor use. The applicability of this finding to patients not on dialysis with ACE inhibitor–associated angioedema is not clear. Although patients with anaphylactoid reactions during dialysis may experience angioedema, these patients typically have hypotension, which is not a feature of ACE inhibitor–associated angioedema. In addition, membrane APP is encoded for by an X-linked gene, but ACE inhibitor–associated angioedema is more common in women than in men. A subsequent study found that the -2399A allele is associated with decreased plasma APP activity in both men and women, but the variant allele is associated with ACE inhibitor–associated angioedema only in men.[34]

Neprilysin also degrades bradykinin and substance P. Pare and colleagues[35] reported an association between a polymorphism in the gene encoding neprilysin and ACE inhibitor–associated angioedema of African American ancestry in a case-control study in Tennessee as well as in the Ongoing Telmisartan Alone and in Combination with Ramipril Global Endpoint Trial (ONTARGET). The investigators also conducted a genome-wide association study in 175 individuals with ACE inhibitor–associated angioedema and 489 ACE inhibitor–exposed controls without angioedema from Nashville (Tennessee) and Marshfield (Wisconsin). No associations of genome-wide significance were found. Of the SNPs that were associated modestly with ACE inhibitor–associated angioedema in the Nashville/Marshfield analysis, 2 were also significantly associated with ACE inhibitor–associated angioedema (rs500766 and rs2724635) in ONTARGET cases versus controls. Rs500766 is a polymorphism in the gene encoding protein kinase C θ (PRKCQ). In both the Nashville/Marshfield sample (odds ratio [OR], 0.42; 95% confidence interval [CI], 0.28–0.63; $P = 2.97 \times 10^{-5}$ in the additive model: OR, 0.42; 95% CI, 0.26–0.67; $P = 3.04 \times 10^{-4}$ in the dominant model) and in ONTARGET (OR, 0.28; 95% CI, 0.09–0.89; $P = .03$ in the dominant genetic model), the T allele was significantly associated with a reduced risk of ACE inhibitor–associated angioedema. Rs2724635 is a polymorphism in ETS variant gene 6 (ETV6), also known as TEL (translocation ets leukemia), and the G allele was associated with an increased risk of ACE inhibitor–associated angioedema in both African Americans in the Nashville/Marshfield sample (OR, 2.78; 95% CI, 1.67–4.00; $P = 2.73 \times 10^{-5}$ in the additive model; OR, 3.23; 95% CI, 1.75–6.25; $P = 2.11 \times 10^{-4}$ in the dominant model; OR, 5.56; 95% CI, 1.85–16.6; $P = 2.01 \times 10^{-3}$ in the recessive model) and in the ONTARGET sample (OR, 3.27; 95% CI, 1.03–10.35; $P = .044$ recessive model). Both of these genes are involved in immune regulation and their association with ACE inhibitor–associated angioedema is intriguing given the clinical association of ACE inhibitor–associated angioedema with seasonal allergies and with immunosuppressant use.

Management of Angiotensin-converting Enzyme Inhibitor–associated Angioedema

The mainstays of the management of ACE inhibitor–associated angioedema remain recognition, discontinuation of the ACE inhibitor, and airway management. A question that often arises is whether patients who have had ACE inhibitor–associated angioedema can take an angiotensin receptor blocker (ARB) safely. Several studies suggest that it is safe to treat patients with a history of ACE inhibitor–associated angioedema with an ARB. In the Telmisartan Randomized Assessment in ACE Intolerant Subjects with Cardiovascular Disease (TRANSCEND) trial, 2 of 2954 patients (0.07%) randomized to telmisartan had angioedema and 3 of 2972 (0.1%) receiving placebo experienced angioedema.[36] In case-control or cohort studies, the risk of angioedema in ARB users is similar to that in the general population and significantly decreased compared with the rate of angioedema in ACE inhibitor users.[37,38] On this basis, ARBs may be tried in patients who require interruption of the renin-angiotensin system. Because tissue ACE may be inhibited for up to 3 weeks after discontinuation of an ACE inhibitor and angioedema can recur during this period, it is recommended that clinicians allow 6 weeks before any trial of an ARB. Delayed recurrences beyond 6 weeks should raise the suspicion of another cause of angioedema.

The selective B_2 antagonist icatibant (D-Arg-[Hyp3, Thi5, D-Tic7, Oic8]-bradykinin) reduces the time to resolution of symptoms in patients with hereditary angioedema and has been approved by the US Food and Drug Administration (FDA) for treatment of hereditary angioedema.[39,40] Three randomized clinical studies have assessed the effect of B_2 receptor antagonism in ACE inhibitor–associated angioedema.[41] The first, a small multicenter study conducted in Germany, reported that icatibant reduced the time to complete resolution of ACE inhibitor–associated angioedema in patients of European descent.[41] A second small study conducted in a single center in the United States did not find any effect of icatibant on the time to resolution of symptoms, or the severity of symptoms in patients with ACE inhibitor–associated angioedema.[42] A third study, a multicenter study in 120 patients with ACE inhibitor–associated angioedema, also did not find an effect of the B_2 receptor antagonist icatibant on the time to discharge (Sinert and colleagues, *Academic Emerg Med* 2016 abstract).

The Bas and colleagues[41] trial differed from the 2 studies showing no effect of icatibant in ACE inhibitor–associated angioedema in several important ways. In the Bas and colleagues[41] study, assessment of injection site reactions might have inadvertently resulted in unblinding. The study used an active comparator rather than placebo control. All of the patients were white and 62% were male, whereas ACE inhibitor–associated angioedema is more common among African Americans and women; these two groups were more prevalent in the negative clinical studies. Based on the lack of definitive evidence to support a benefit of B_2 receptor antagonism in ACE inhibitor–associated angioedema, icatibant is not approved for this indication.

The lack of effect of bradykinin B_2 receptor antagonism on symptoms in patients with ACE inhibitor–associated angioedema contrasts with the efficacy of B_2 receptor antagonism in hereditary angioedema.[39,40] Likewise, ecallantide, a kallikrein inhibitor approved for the treatment of hereditary angioedema, is not effective in ACE inhibitor–associated angioedema.[43,44] These findings suggest that substance P or other peptide substrates of ACE inhibitors can contribute to and perpetuate angioedema even when the B_2 receptor is blocked. Delay in treatment could also reduce the efficacy of B_2 receptor antagonism in patients with ACE inhibitor–associated angioedema. The mean time from the onset of symptoms to study drug administration ranged from 6.1 to 10.3 hours in clinical trials of icatibant in ACE inhibitor–associated angioedema.[41,42]

DIPEPTIDYL PEPTIDASE 4 INHIBITORS AND ANGIOEDEMA

In recent years, new classes of drugs that decrease the degradation of vasoactive peptides implicated in the pathogenesis of angioedema have been approved. Dipeptidyl peptidase 4 (DPP4) cleaves the amino terminus dipeptide from peptides with a proline or alanine as the penultimate amino acids, including the incretins glucagonlike peptide-1 and glucose-dependent insulinotropic polypeptide. By decreasing the degradation of incretins, DPP4 inhibitors, approved for the treatment of diabetes, increase insulin secretion in a glucose-dependent manner, decrease appetite, and suppress glucose-dependent glucagon secretion.

Substance P is a substrate of both ACE and DPP4. Brown and colleagues[45] reported that concurrent DPP4 inhibitor use increases the risk of ACE inhibitor–associated angioedema. In the Saxagliptin Assessment of Vascular Outcomes Recorded in patients with diabetes mellitus–Thrombolysis in Myocardial Infarction (SAVOR-TIMI) 53 study, saxagliptin treatment was associated with an increased incidence of angioedema compared with placebo treatment (8 vs 1; $P = .04$),[46] which is an incidence of $\sim 0.1\%$. The incidence of angioedema in other clinical trials of DPP4 inhibitors is often hard to discern because angioedema is conflated with hypersensitivity reactions.

COMBINED ANGIOTENSIN RECEPTOR BLOCKER/NEPRILYSIN INHIBITOR AND ANGIOEDEMA

Neprilysin degrades bradykinin and substance P, as well as natriuretic peptides. In the late twentieth century, a combined ACE/NEP inhibitor, omapatrilat, was developed for the treatment of hypertension and heart failure. Omapatrilat was never approved by the FDA but clinical trials implicated the neprilysin pathway in the pathophysiology of angioedema. In the Omapatrilat Cardiovascular Treatment Versus Enalapril (OCTAVE) double-blind, active-controlled trial in 25,302 patients with untreated or uncontrolled hypertension, the incidence of angioedema was 2.17% in the combined ACE/NEP inhibitor–treated group compared with 0.68% in the enalapril group.[15] The incidence of angioedema was increased in patients of African descent in both the omapatrilat and the enalapril treatment groups.

The increased incidence of angioedema during treatment with omapatrilat compared with enalapril alone has been attributed to the concurrent blockade of 2 pathways involved in the degradation of bradykinin and substance P. Recently, the combined ARB/NEP inhibitor valsartan/sacubitril was approved for the treatment of heart failure based on a beneficial effect on mortality compared with enalapril in the Prospective comparison of ARNI with ACEI to Determine Impact on Global Mortality and Morbidity in Heart Failure (PARADIGM-HF) trial.[17] In this study there were 19 cases of angioedema in the valsartan/sacubitril-treated group (0.45%) compared with 10 in enalapril-treated patients (0.24%). The use of valsartan/sacubitril may lead to a higher incidence of angioedema in clinical practice. In PARADGIM-HF, 77% of the patients enrolled in the trial had been treated previously with an ACE inhibitor and all patients were exposed to an ACE inhibitor during a run-in period.[17] In addition, the number of African Americans studied was small and, as in ACE inhibitor–associated angioedema, the incidence of valsartan/sacubitril-associated angioedema is higher in patients of African ancestry compared with those of European ancestry.

TISSUE-TYPE PLASMINOGEN ACTIVATOR–INDUCED ANGIOEDEMA

Angioedema occurs in 1.3% to 7.9% of patients who are treated with recombinant tissue-type plasminogen activator (tPA) for ischemic stroke.[47,48] In contrast, angioedema occurs rarely (0.02%) in patients given tPA in the treatment of myocardial infarction.[48] ACE inhibitor use is associated with a significantly increased risk of angioedema following recombinant tPA,[47–49] suggesting that tPA administration leads to the production of a vasoactive ACE substrate. Molinaro and colleagues[50] reported that incubation of plasma with microgram-per-milliliter t-PA in the presence of the ACE inhibitor enalaprilat results in the generation of bradykinin. Bradykinin generation depended on the activation of plasminogen to plasmin, and subsequent activation of the contact system.

SUMMARY

Angioedema associated with medications can occur via bradykinin-mediated, histamine-mediated, or leukotriene-mediated mechanisms. A growing number of drugs may cause angioedema via bradykinin. The mainstay in treatment of nonallergic drug-induced angioedema is cessation of the offending agents.

REFERENCES

1. Jares EJ, Sanchez-Borges M, Cardona-Villa R, et al. Multinational experience with hypersensitivity drug reactions in Latin America. Ann Allergy Asthma Immunol 2014;113(3):282–9.
2. Bertazzoni G, Spina MT, Scarpellini MG, et al. Drug-induced angioedema: experience of Italian emergency departments. Intern Emerg Med 2014;9(4):455–62.
3. Banerji A, Oren E, Hesterberg P, et al. Ten-year study of causes of moderate to severe angioedema seen by an inpatient allergy/immunology consult service. Allergy Asthma Proc 2008;29:88–92.
4. Kowalski ML, Woessner K, Sanak M. Approaches to the diagnosis and management of patients with a history of nonsteroidal anti-inflammatory drug-related urticaria and angioedema. J Allergy Clin Immunol 2015;136(2):245–51.
5. Kowalski ML, Bienkiewicz B, Woszczek G, et al. Diagnosis of pyrazolone drug sensitivity: clinical history versus skin testing and in vitro testing. Allergy Asthma Proc 1999;20(6):347–52.
6. Cornejo-Garcia JA, Jagemann LR, Blanca-Lopez N, et al. Genetic variants of the arachidonic acid pathway in non-steroidal anti-inflammatory drug-induced acute urticaria. Clin Exp Allergy 2012;42(12):1772–81.

7. Plaza-Seron Mdel C, Ayuso P, Perez-Sanchez N, et al. Copy number variation in ALOX5 and PTGER1 is associated with NSAIDs-induced urticaria and/or angioedema. Pharmacogenet Genomics 2016;26(6):280–7.

8. Oussalah A, Mayorga C, Blanca M, et al. Genetic variants associated with drugs-induced immediate hypersensitivity reactions: a PRISMA-compliant systematic review. Allergy 2016;71(4):443–62.

9. Wong JT, Nagy CS, Krinzman SJ, et al. Rapid oral challenge-desensitization for patients with aspirin-related urticaria-angioedema. J Allergy Clin Immunol 2000; 105(5):997–1001.

10. Mahmoudpour SH, Baranova EV, Souverein PC, et al. Determinants of angiotensin-converting enzyme inhibitor (ACEI) intolerance and angioedema in the UK Clinical Practice Research Datalink. Br J Clin Pharmacol 2016;82(6): 1647–59.

11. Brown NJ, Snowden M, Griffin MR. Recurrent angiotensin-converting enzyme inhibitor–associated angioedema. JAMA 1997;278(3):232–3.

12. Miller DR, Oliveria SA, Berlowitz DR, et al. Angioedema incidence in US veterans initiating angiotensin-converting enzyme inhibitors. Hypertension 2008;51(6): 1624–30.

13. Kieu MC, Bangiyev JN, Thottam PJ, et al. Predictors of airway intervention in angiotensin-converting enzyme inhibitor-induced angioedema. Otolaryngol Head Neck Surg 2015;153(4):544–50.

14. Slater EE, Merrill DD, Guess HA, et al. Clinical profile of angioedema associated with angiotensin converting-enzyme inhibition. JAMA 1988;260(7):967–70.

15. Kostis JB, Packer M, Black HR, et al. Omapatrilat and enalapril in patients with hypertension: the Omapatrilat Cardiovascular Treatment vs. Enalapril (OCTAVE) trial. Am J Hypertens 2004;17(2):103–11.

16. Sica DA. The African American Study of Kidney Disease and Hypertension (AASK) trial: what more have we learned? J Clin Hypertens (Greenwich) 2003; 5(2):159–67.

17. McMurray JJ, Packer M, Desai AS, et al. Angiotensin-neprilysin inhibition versus enalapril in heart failure. N Engl J Med 2014;371(11):993–1004.

18. Brown NJ, Ray WA, Snowden M, et al. Black Americans have an increased rate of angiotensin converting enzyme inhibitor-associated angioedema. Clin Pharmacol Ther 1996;60(1):8–13.

19. Gibbs CR, Lip GY, Beevers DG. Angioedema due to ACE inhibitors: increased risk in patients of African origin. Br J Clin Pharmacol 1999;48(6):861–5.

20. Kostis JB, Kim HJ, Rusnak J, et al. Incidence and characteristics of angioedema associated with enalapril. Arch Intern Med 2005;165(14):1637–42.

21. Straka B, Nian H, Sloan C, et al. Pollen count and presentation of angiotensin-converting enzyme inhibitor-associated angioedema. J Allergy Clin Immunol Pract 2013;1(5):468–73.e1-4.

22. Abbosh J, Anderson JA, Levine AB, et al. Angiotensin converting enzyme inhibitor-induced angioedema more prevalent in transplant patients. Ann Allergy Asthma Immunol 1999;82(5):473–6.

23. Byrd JB, Woodard-Grice A, Stone E, et al. Association of angiotensin-converting enzyme inhibitor-associated angioedema with transplant and immunosuppressant use. Allergy 2010;65(11):1381–7.

24. Zuraw BL. Clinical practice. Hereditary angioedema. N Engl J Med 2008;359(10): 1027–36.

25. de Oliveira JR, Otuki MF, Cabrini DA, et al. Involvement of the TRPV1 receptor in plasma extravasation in airways of rats treated with an angiotensin-converting enzyme inhibitor. Pulm Pharmacol Ther 2016;41:25–33.

26. Sulpizio AC, Pullen MA, Edwards RM, et al. The effect of acute angiotensin-converting enzyme and neutral endopeptidase 24.11 inhibition on plasma extravasation in the rat. J Pharmacol Exp Ther 2004;309(3):1141–7.

27. Emanueli C, Grady EF, Madeddu P, et al. Acute ACE inhibition causes plasma extravasation in mice that is mediated by bradykinin and substance P. Hypertension 1998;31(6):1299–304.

28. Byrd JB, Shreevatsa A, Putlur P, et al. Dipeptidyl peptidase IV deficiency increases susceptibility to angiotensin-converting enzyme inhibitor-induced peritracheal edema. J Allergy Clin Immunol 2007;120(2):403–8.

29. Moholisa RR, Rayner BR, Patricia Owen E, et al. Association of B2 receptor polymorphisms and ACE activity with ACE inhibitor-induced angioedema in black and mixed-race South Africans. J Clin Hypertens (Greenwich) 2013;15(6):413–9.

30. Lung CC, Chan EK, Zuraw BL. Analysis of an exon 1 polymorphism of the B2 bradykinin receptor gene and its transcript in normal subjects and patients with C1 inhibitor deficiency. J Allergy Clin Immunol 1997;99(1 Pt 1):134–46.

31. Bas M, Hoffmann TK, Tiemann B, et al. Potential genetic risk factors in angiotensin-converting enzyme-inhibitor-induced angio-oedema. Br J Clin Pharmacol 2010;69(2):179–86.

32. Gulec M, Caliskaner Z, Tunca Y, et al. The role of ace gene polymorphism in the development of angioedema secondary to angiotensin converting enzyme inhibitors and angiotensin II receptor blockers. Allergol Immunopathol (Madr) 2008; 36(3):134–40.

33. Duan QL, Nikpoor B, Dube MP, et al. A variant in XPNPEP2 is associated with angioedema induced by angiotensin I-converting enzyme inhibitors. Am J Hum Genet 2005;77(4):617–26.

34. Woodard-Grice AV, Lucisano AC, Byrd JB, et al. Sex-dependent and race-dependent association of XPNPEP2 C-2399A polymorphism with angiotensin-converting enzyme inhibitor-associated angioedema. Pharmacogenet Genomics 2010;20(9):532–6.

35. Pare G, Kubo M, Byrd JB, et al. Genetic variants associated with angiotensin-converting enzyme inhibitor-associated angioedema. Pharmacogenet Genomics 2013;23(9):470–8.

36. Telmisartan Randomised AssessmeNt Study in ACE iNtolerant subjects with cardiovascular Disease (TRANSCEND) Investigators, Yusuf S, Teo K, Anderson C, et al. Effects of the angiotensin-receptor blocker telmisartan on cardiovascular events in high-risk patients intolerant to angiotensin-converting enzyme inhibitors: a randomised controlled trial. Lancet 2008;372(9644):1174–83.

37. Johnsen SP, Jacobsen J, Monster TB, et al. Risk of first-time hospitalization for angioedema among users of ACE inhibitors and angiotensin receptor antagonists. Am J Med 2005;118(12):1428–9.

38. Toh S, Reichman ME, Houstoun M, et al. Comparative risk for angioedema associated with the use of drugs that target the renin-angiotensin-aldosterone system. Arch Intern Med 2012;172(20):1582–9.

39. Cicardi M, Banerji A, Bracho F, et al. Icatibant, a new bradykinin-receptor antagonist, in hereditary angioedema. N Engl J Med 2010;363(6):532–41.

40. Lumry WR, Li HH, Levy RJ, et al. Randomized placebo-controlled trial of the bradykinin B(2) receptor antagonist icatibant for the treatment of acute attacks of

hereditary angioedema: the FAST-3 trial. Ann Allergy Asthma Immunol 2011; 107(6):529–37.

41. Bas M, Greve J, Stelter K, et al. A randomized trial of icatibant in ACE-inhibitor-induced angioedema. N Engl J Med 2015;372(5):418–25.

42. Straka BT, Ramirez CE, Byrd JB, et al. Effect of bradykinin receptor antagonism on ACE inhibitor-associated angioedema. J Allergy Clin Immunol 2016. [Epub ahead of print].

43. Lewis LM, Graffeo C, Crosley P, et al. Ecallantide for the acute treatment of angiotensin-converting enzyme inhibitor-induced angioedema: a multicenter, randomized, controlled trial. Ann Emerg Med 2015;65(2):204–13.

44. Bernstein JA, Moellman JJ, Collins SP, et al. Effectiveness of ecallantide in treating angiotensin-converting enzyme inhibitor-induced angioedema in the emergency department. Ann Allergy Asthma Immunol 2015;114(3):245–9.

45. Brown NJ, Byiers S, Carr D, et al. Dipeptidyl peptidase-IV inhibitor use associated with increased risk of ACE inhibitor-associated angioedema. Hypertension 2009; 54(3):516–23.

46. Scirica BM, Bhatt DL, Braunwald E, et al. Saxagliptin and cardiovascular outcomes in patients with type 2 diabetes mellitus. N Engl J Med 2013;369(14): 1317–26.

47. Hill MD, Buchan AM, Canadian Alteplase for Stroke Effectiveness Study (CASES) Investigators. Thrombolysis for acute ischemic stroke: results of the Canadian Alteplase for Stroke Effectiveness Study. CMAJ 2005;172(10):1307–12.

48. Hurford R, Rezvani S, Kreimei M, et al. Incidence, predictors and clinical characteristics of orolingual angio-oedema complicating thrombolysis with tissue plasminogen activator for ischaemic stroke. J Neurol Neurosurg Psychiatry 2015; 86(5):520–3.

49. Lin SY, Tang SC, Tsai LK, et al. Orolingual angioedema after alteplase therapy of acute ischaemic stroke: incidence and risk of prior angiotensin-converting enzyme inhibitor use. Eur J Neurol 2014;21(10):1285–91.

50. Molinaro G, Gervais N, Adam A. Biochemical basis of angioedema associated with recombinant tissue plasminogen activator treatment: an in vitro experimental approach. Stroke 2002;33(6):1712–6.

51. Thong B. Update on the management of antibiotic allergy. Allergy Asthma Immunol Res 2010;2(2):77–86.

52. Perez-Inestrosa E, Suau R, Montanez M, et al. Cephalosporin chemical reactivity and its immunological implications. Curr Opin Allergy Clin Immunol 2005;5(4): 323–30.

53. Manfredi M, Severino M, Testi S, et al. Detection of specific IgE to quinolones. J Allergy Clin Immunol 2004;113(1):155–60.

54. Gruchalla R, Sullivan T. Detection of human IgE to sulfamethoxazole by skin testing with sulfamethoxazoyl-poly-L-tyrosine. J Allergy Clin Immunol 1991; 88(5):784–92.

55. Wong J, Ripple R, MacLean J, et al. Vancomycin hypersensitivity: synergism with narcotics and "desensitization" by a rapid continuous intravenous protocol. J Allergy Clin Immunol 1994;94(2 pt 1):189–94.

56. Araújo L, Demoly P. Macrolides allergy. Curr Pharm Des 2008;14(27):2840–62.

57. Markman M, Kennedy A, Webster K, et al. Clinical features of hypersensitivity reactions to carboplatin. J Clin Oncol 1999;17(4):1141.

58. Markman M, Kennedy A, Webster K, et al. Paclitaxel-associated hypersensitivity reactions: experience of the gynecologic oncology program of the Cleveland Clinic Cancer Center. J Clin Oncol 2000;18(1):102–5.

59. Chung C, Mirahkur B, Chan E, et al. Cetuximab-induced anaphylaxis and IgE specific for galactose-alpha-1,3-galactose. N Engl J Med 2008;358(11):1109–17.

60. Lerondeau B, Trechot P, Waton J, et al. Analysis of cross-reactivity among radiocontrast media in 97 hypersensitivity reactions. J Allergy Clin Immunol 2016; 137(2):633–5.e4.

61. Harle D, Baldo B, Coroneos N, et al. Anaphylaxis following administration of papaveretum. Implications of IgE antibodies that react with morphine and codeine, and identification of an allergic determinant. Anesthesiology 1989;71(4):489–94.

62. Mertes P, Volcheck G, Garvey L, et al. Epidemiology of perioperative anaphylaxis. La Presse Médicale 2016;45(9):758–67.

63. Giavina-Bianchi P, Aun M, Jares E, et al. Angioedema associated with nonsteroidal anti-inflammatory drugs. Curr Opin Allergy Clin Immunol 2016;16:323–32.

64. Chang Y. Hypersensitivity reactions to proton pump inhibitors. Curr Opin Allergy Clin Immunol 2012;12(4):348–53.

65. Wenande E, Garvey L. Immediate-type hypersensitivity to polyethylene glycols: a review. Clin Exp Allergy 2016;46(7):907–22.

66. Subramanian H, Gupta K, Ali H. Roles of Mas-related G protein-coupled receptor X2 on mast cell-mediated host defense, pseudoallergic drug reactions, and chronic inflammatory diseases. J Allergy Clin Immunol 2016;138(3):700–10.

67. Joint Task Force on Practice Parameters, American Academy of Allergy, Asthma and Immunology, American College of Allergy, Asthma and Immunology, Joint Council of Allergy, Asthma and Immunology. Drug allergy: an updated practice parameter. Ann Allergy Asthma Immunol 2015;105(4):259–73.

68. Eisenhauer E, ten Bokkel Huinink W, Swenerton K, et al. European-Canadian randomized trial of paclitaxel in relapsed ovarian cancer: high-dose versus low-dose and long versus short infusion. J Clin Oncol 1994;12(12):2654–66.

69. Brockow K. Immediate and delayed cutaneous reactions to radiocontrast media. Chem Immunol Allergy 2012;97:180–90.

70. Solinski H, Gudermann T, Breit A. Pharmacology and signaling of Mas-related G protein-coupled receptors. Pharmacol Rev 2014;66(3):570–97.

71. Gisler V, Müller S, Müller L, et al. Acute angioedema triggered by daptomycin. Infect Dis Ther 2016;5(2):201–5.

72. Lammintausta K, Tokola R, Kalimo K. Cutaneous adverse reactions to clindamycin: results of tests and oral exposure. Br J Dermatol 2001;146:643–8.

73. Palchick B, Funk E, McEntire J, et al. Anaphylaxis due to chloramphenicol. Am J Med Sci 1984;288:43–5.

74. Buergin S, Scherer K, Häusermann P, et al. Immediate hypersensitivity to rifampicin in 3 patients: diagnostic procedures and induction of clinical tolerance. Int Arch Allergy Immunol 2006;140(1):20–6.

75. Iikura M, Yamaguchi M, Hirai K, et al. Case report: streptomycin-induced anaphylactic shock during oocyte retrieval process for in vitro fertilization. J Allergy Clin Immunol 2002;109:571–2.

76. Wong P, Yew W, Wong C, et al. Ethambutol-induced pulmonary infiltrates with eosinophilia and skin involvement. Eur Respir J 1995;8(5):866–8.

77. Crook M. Isoniazid-induced anaphylaxis. Clin Pharmacol 2003;43(5):545–6.

78. Lykavieris P, Frauger E, Habes D, et al. Angioedema in pediatric liver transplant recipients under tacrolimus immunosuppression. Transplantation 2003;75(1): 152–5.

79. Wadei H, Gruber S, El-Amm J, et al. Sirolimus-induced angioedema. Am J Transplant 2004;4(6):1002–5.

80. Krasowska D, Szymanek M, Schwartz R, et al. Cutaneous effects of the most commonly used antidepressant medication, the selective serotonin reuptake inhibitors. J Am Acad Dermatol 2007;56(5):848–53.
81. Eberhart A, Weiler C, Erie J. Angioedema related to the use of hyaluronidase in cataract surgery. Am J Ophthalmol 2004;138(1):142–3.

Acquired C1 Inhibitor Deficiency

Iris M. Otani, MD[a],*, Aleena Banerji, MD[b]

KEYWORDS

- Acquired angioedema • C1 esterase inhibitor deficiency • Rituximab
- Lymphoproliferative disorders • Anti-C1 esterase inhibitor autoantibody

KEY POINTS

- Acquired angioedema with C1-INH deficiency (C1-INH-AAE) should be considered when patients present with isolated angioedema without urticaria in the fourth decade of life or later without a family history of angioedema.
- A quantitative or functional C1-INH deficiency with negative family history and low C1q is diagnostic of C1-INH-AAE.
- All patients diagnosed with C1-INH-AAE should be evaluated for an underlying B-cell lymphoproliferative disorder at the time of diagnosis. If no disorder is found, repeat evaluation annually is recommended. A diagnosis of C1-INH-AAE can precede a diagnosis of lymphoproliferative disease and confers an increased risk for developing non-Hodgkin lymphoma.
- Treatment focuses on symptom control with therapies that regulate bradykinin activity (C1-INH concentrate, icatibant, ecallantide, tranexamic acid, androgens) and treatment of any underlying conditions.
- Rituximab has been used successfully to treat C1-INH-AAE.

INTRODUCTION

Angioedema is defined as transient localized swelling of the subcutaneous and/or mucosal tissues that can occur anywhere in the body and last for several days. The underlying cause of angioedema is not easily recognizable on clinical presentation. As angioedema can potentially be fatal, timely identification of the underlying cause is a critical step in ensuring effective treatments are administered for subsequent angioedema attacks.

Disclosures: The authors have no relevant commercial or financial conflicts of interest to disclose.
[a] Department of Medicine, Division of Pulmonary, Allergy, Critical Care, and Sleep Medicine, UCSF Medical Center, 400 Parnassus Avenue, Box 0359, San Francisco, CA 94143, USA;
[b] Department of Medicine, Division of Rheumatology, Allergy and Immunology, Massachusetts General Hospital, Cox 201 Allergy Associates, Boston, MA 02114, USA
* Corresponding author.
E-mail address: iris.otani@ucsf.edu

Immunol Allergy Clin N Am 37 (2017) 497–511
http://dx.doi.org/10.1016/j.iac.2017.03.002
0889-8561/17/© 2017 Elsevier Inc. All rights reserved.

immunology.theclinics.com

When angioedema without urticaria does not either respond to high-dose antihistamines or recur reproducibly after exposure to a specific drug or food, bradykinin-mediated causes should be considered. Angioedema that presents as nonpruritic, nonpitting swelling without urticaria lasting for 2 to 5 days is often considered to be mediated by bradykinin or the release of a vasoactive substance from mast cells and/or basophils.

Angioedema due to C1 esterase inhibitor (C1-INH) deficiency is one of the main causes of bradykinin-mediated angioedema. Testing for C1-INH deficiency is performed by measuring C1-INH antigen level, C1-INH function, and C4 levels in plasma. C1-INH deficiency can be due to a genetic defect (hereditary angioedema, HAE) or an acquired defect (acquired angioedema).

Acquired angioedema was first described by Caldwell and colleagues in 1972.[1] They described a 49-year-old patient with recurrent episodes of angioedema in the setting of lymphosarcoma and C1 inhibitor deficiency. The clinical presentation in this case was indistinguishable from HAE. Further review and evaluation defined the syndrome of acquired angioedema with 3 key elements:

1. Acquired deficiency of C1-INH,
2. Hyperactivation of the classic pathway of human complement, and
3. Recurrent angioedema symptoms.[1]

This condition is now referred to as acquired angioedema due to C1-INH deficiency (C1-INH-AAE). C1-INH-AAE is considered a subset of acquired angioedema, which more broadly includes other conditions such as angiotensin-converting-enzyme inhibitor (ACEI)–associated angioedema.

Although angioedema can be caused by many factors, bradykinin-mediated forms of angioedema are potentially life-threatening conditions, and therefore, appropriate diagnosis and management are critical. In this article, the authors specifically review the literature regarding C1-INH-AAE. This article reviews the epidemiology, risk factors, and clinical presentation of C1-INH-AAE and discusses the approaches to its diagnosis and treatment.

EPIDEMIOLOGY

C1-INH-AAE is a very rare disorder, and only several hundred cases have been reported in the literature to date. Experts in the field estimate that its prevalence may be between 1:100,000 and 1:500,000, based on their experience of identifying one C1-INH-AAE patient for every 10 HAE patients.[2,3] In the group of patients referred to a specialty center in Milan for angioedema due to C1 inhibitor deficiency since 1976, 77 had acquired and 675 had hereditary forms of the disease with a ratio of 1:8.8.[3,4] A 2010 literature review identified 168 probable cases.[5] Two national series in the United Kingdom and Denmark found that between 6% and 10% of angioedema cases were attributable to C1-INH-AAE.[6,7] Because the condition is so often overlooked, the actual prevalence is thought to likely be much higher.[8] In addition, recent data suggest an average lag of 5 years from initial symptoms to diagnosis of C1-INH-AAE.[6]

There are several factors that may contribute to this, as previously described by Cicardi and colleagues[2]:

1. Awareness of C1-INH-AAE is not widespread, and uncertainties regarding the pathogenesis and laboratory features of the disorder further complicate diagnosis.
2. There is no family history of swelling in C1-INH-AAE, so cases are often not detected through family screenings (distinct from HAE).

3. The diagnosis of a coexisting lymphoproliferative malignancy can overshadow other medical issues, including recurrent angioedema, which may be attributed to a paraneoplastic phenomenon and not evaluated further.
4. Because the disorder begins later in life, many patients are taking multiple medications, and the episodes of angioedema are attributed to other causes such as drug reactions. Accordingly, patients may have multiple comorbidities, and the evaluation of angioedema may not take precedence until a severe attack occurs.
5. Complement abnormalities may fluctuate between normal and abnormal when the disorder first develops, becoming more consistently abnormal over the ensuing months. For this reason, mild abnormalities associated with a consistent clinical presentation should be followed over time.

RISK FACTORS

The most common causes of C1-INH-AAE are B-cell lymphoproliferative disorders and autoimmunity. The lymphoproliferative disorders range from monoclonal gammopathies of undetermined significance (MGUS) to B-cell malignancies. Approximately 35% of patients with C1-INH-AAE have MGUS. A recent review identified indolent lymphoma, especially splenic marginal zone lymphoma, and MGUS as the most common conditions associated with C1-INH-AAE.[9] Other conditions associated with C1-INH-AAE include the human immunodeficiency virus, multiple myeloma, Waldenström macroglobulinemia, systemic lupus erythematosus, Churg-Strauss syndrome, xanthomatosis, and hepatitis B and other infections.

Overall, approximately 70% of patients with C1-INH-AAE are found to have an associated disorder.[10] In half of these cases, the disorder is malignant (most often non-Hodgkin lymphomas [NHL]), and in the other half, the associated condition is benign (MGUS).[2]

CLINICAL FEATURES

The clinical presentation of C1-INH-AAE is difficult to distinguish clinically from HAE type 1 and 2 except that a family history is lacking and angioedema generally develops after the age of 40 years. Persons of any race or gender can be affected equally by C1-INH-AAE. Angioedema in C1-INH-AAE patients occurs in cutaneous and mucosal tissues and can involve any part of the body, but often presents as swelling of the face, lips, tongue, larynx, or extremities. Swelling episodes occur without urticaria and typically resolve within 2 to 5 days. Attacks are commonly triggered by stress, trauma, and viral infections, but often occur without an identifiable trigger.[11]

Compared with urticarial swelling, the swelling of angioedema is deeper and longer lasting, is nonpruritic, and may be painful.[12] Angioedema may involve the gastrointestinal tract, leading to intestinal wall edema, which results in symptoms such as abdominal pain, nausea, vomiting, and diarrhea. Facial edema and abdominal pain were the most frequent symptoms reported in C1-INH-AAE patients.[9] C1-INH-AAE can be life threatening, and acute laryngeal edema is the major cause of angioedema-related mortality. Around 50% of patients with C1-INH-AAE experience upper airway edema, and anoxic brain injury or death from upper airway obstruction can occur.[13,14]

There are other more subtle differences between the clinical manifestations of the C1-INH-AAE and HAE described by Cicardi[2]:

1. Gastrointestinal attacks presenting as recurrent colicky abdominal pain, distention, vomiting, and/or diarrhea are less common in C1-INH-AAE compared with HAE. These types of attacks are reported by nearly 80% of patients with HAE type 1

and 2, whereas less than 50% of C1-INH-AAE reported gastrointestinal attacks.[13,15]

2. In C1-INH-AAE, angioedema seems to affect the face more than the extremities, which is distinctly opposite from patients with HAE type 1 and 2, where swelling of the extremities is more typical.[13] However, both disorders can cause swellings in the face and extremities.

3. Patients may describe a prodrome of erythema marginatum before cutaneous or gastrointestinal angioedema episodes, but it is extremely rare especially when compared with patients with HAE type 1 and 2.

C1-INH-AAE should be considered in a patient who presents with isolated angioedema (without urticaria) in the fourth decade of life or later without a family history of angioedema. All patients with C1-INH-AAE should be evaluated for an underlying B-cell lymphoproliferative disorder at the time of diagnosis. If no disorder is found, repeat evaluation annually is recommended.

PATHOPHYSIOLOGY

C1-INH is a serine protease inhibitor that inhibits C1r and C1s in the classical complement system, production of FXIIa and kallikrein in the kallikrein-kinin system, and FXIa in the kallikrein-kinin and coagulation systems.[16,17] C1-INH controls bradykinin generation via its inhibitory effects on FXIIa and kallikrein. Angioedema due to deficiency or dysfunction of C1-INH is mediated by the binding of bradykinin to bradykinin B2 receptors on endothelial cells.[16]

When there is a deficiency of the C1-INH protein, overactivation of the kallikrein-kinin system leads to bradykinin production. Inactive FXII and plasma prekallikrein are cleaved to their active forms FXIIa and kallikrein, respectively. Activated kallikrein cleaves high-molecular-weight kininogen to release bradykinin.[16–18] Bradykinin binds to bradykinin B2 receptors on endothelial cells, leading to nitric oxide production, relaxation of the smooth muscle in the vessel wall, and increased vascular permeability.[16,19] Vasodilation, increased vascular permeability, and localized fluid extravasation result in angioedema.[16,20]

Acquired angioedema due to deficiency of C1-INH, or C1-INH-AAE, occurs when there are acquired (not inherited) deficiencies of C1-INH. Although the exact pathophysiology is unclear, evidence suggests that there are 2 major mechanisms that can cause a C1-INH–deficient state in C1-INH-AAE:

1. Overconsumption of C1-INH by neoplastic lymphatic tissue and
2. The production of anti-C1-INH autoantibodies.[16,17,20,21]

As such, C1-INH-AAE has historically been classified into type I (absence of C1-INH autoantibodies) and type II (presence of C1-INH autoantibodies).[22]

Initially, it was thought that malignant lymphoproliferation and autoimmunity were uniquely responsible for the 2 types of C1-INH-AAE: type I (paraneoplastic overconsumption of C1-INH) and type II (autoimmune production of anti-C1-INH autoantibodies).[10] It was thought that lymphoproliferation and autoimmunity were uniquely responsible for Type I and Type II C1-INH-AAE because initial cases of C1-INH-AAE were reported in association with lymphoproliferative disease,[23–28] and there was evidence that C1-INH reduction was due to consumption by lymphatic tissue. Hauptmann and colleagues[29] investigated the properties of splenic lymphosarcoma tissue resected from a patient with AAE and splenic lymphosarcoma and demonstrated that in vitro incubation of lymphosarcoma tissue with guinea pig serum led to complement depletion. Schreiber and colleagues[23] also investigated the properties of lymphoid tissue from a patient with AAE and B-cell lymphoproliferative disorder with lymphoid cells infiltrating the pulmonary parenchyma and found that in vitro incubation of lung biopsy tissue with human serum led to complement depletion. Geha and colleagues[30] found evidence that the mechanism of C1-INH consumption in B-cell lymphoproliferative disorders was due to the formation of idiotype/anti-idiotype immune complexes. The discovery of an autoreactive immunoglobulin G against C1-INH by Jackson and colleagues[31] provided evidence that some cases of C1-INH-AAE could have an autoimmune basis.

Taken together, these cases supported a hypothesis that in type I AAE, malignant lymphoproliferation led to C1-INH overconsumption, and that in type II AAE, autoimmune production of anti-C1-INH autoantibodies led to inadequate C1-INH function.

However, subsequent reports have shown that the pathophysiology is not so clear. B-cell lymphoproliferative disorders were found to be equally prevalent in both type I and type II AAE, and monoclonal paraproteinemia can account for anti-C1-INH autoantibody production. On the other hand, anti-C1-INH autoantibodies are present in AAE patients both with and without underlying B-cell lymphoproliferative disorders, indicating that monoclonal B-cell lymphoproliferation is not the sole mechanism for anti-C1-INH autoantibody production.[10,32]

In a case series of 42 patients with AAE, 21 patients had B-cell lymphoproliferative disorders (LPD) and anti-C1-INH autoantibodies, 11 patients had anti-C1-INH autoantibodies with no evidence of B-cell LPD, and 10 patients had B-cell LPD without anti-C1-INH autoantibodies.[10]

In another case series of 13 patients with AAE, anti-C1-INH autoantibody was present in 12 of these 13 patients who did not have a diagnosis of B-cell LPD at time of AAE diagnosis. Seven of these patients were subsequently diagnosed with monoclonal paraproteinemia and 1 patient was subsequently diagnosed with CLL. Although 5 of the 7 patients with an M-component had paraproteins that bound C1-INH, indicating that the paraproteins were anti-C1-INH autoantibodies, 2 patients produced paraproteins that did not bind C1-INH.[32]

These case series in conjunction with cases of patients with C1-INH-AAE and autoimmunity without evidence of anti-C1-INH autoantibodies suggest that the type I and type II classification may be misleading.[10,32–37] This is discussed in more detail in later discussion under Current Controversies.

DIFFERENTIAL DIAGNOSIS

The differential diagnosis for a patient presenting with angioedema is broad. Most causes of angioedema fall into 1 of 2 categories: histamine-mediated or bradykinin-mediated angioedema.[21] Histamine-mediated angioedema (food allergy, drug allergy, stinging insect allergy, chronic idiopathic urticaria and angioedema, mastocytosis, mast cell activation syndromes, idiopathic histaminergic anaphylaxis) is typically associated with urticaria and responds to antihistamines, glucocorticoids, and/or epinephrine.[21,38–44] Suspicion for bradykinin-mediated angioedema is raised when angioedema has the clinical features described in the Clinical Features section above (ie, no pruritus, no hives, no response to antihistamines/epinephrine).[20,21] Angioedema can also be a clinical feature of thyroid dysfunction, Melkersson-Rosenthal syndrome, episodic angioedema with eosinophilia, nonepisodic angioedema with eosinophilia, and disorders causing generalized edema (such as capillary leak syndrome, nephrotic syndrome, cirrhosis, and heart failure).[45–53] Aspirin/nonsteroidal anti-inflammatory drug–induced angioedema due to presumed aberrations in arachidonic acid metabolism can also be seen.[54]

Bradykinin-mediated causes of angioedema include ACEI-induced angioedema due to inadequate bradykinin degradation and hereditary and acquired C1-INH deficiencies due to bradykinin overproduction.[12,38,55] As ACEI-induced angioedema is a clinical diagnosis, a detailed history regarding ACEI use is necessary when evaluating a patient with suspected bradykinin-mediated angioedema. ACEI angioedema can occur over a year after ACEI therapy is initiated and can occur up to 2 months after ACEI therapy is discontinued.[56]

Hereditary and acquired C1-INH deficiencies are associated with alterations in complement levels.[55] Measurements of C4, C1-INH concentration, C1-INH function, and C1q can differentiate between hereditary and acquired C1-INH deficiencies (**Table 1**). Hereditary and acquired angioedema have similar clinical characteristics. However, 90% of patients with HAE present during the first or second decade of life, and most patients with C1-INH-AAE present after the fourth decade of life.[57] Also, HAE with C1-INH deficiency and HAE type II with low C1-INH function are associated with a family inheritance patterns in most cases (~75%), whereas C1-INH-AAE is not.[12,58]

A quantitative or functional C1-INH deficiency with negative family history and low C1q is diagnostic of C1-INH-AAE.[59] C1-INH-AAE is historically classified into type I and type II based on absence and presence of anti-C1-INH autoantibodies, respectively, although this classification system is debated.[22] Only specialized laboratories are able to identify anti-C1-INH autoantibodies.[20]

MANAGEMENT

Management of C1-INH-AAE is aimed at symptom control as well as identification and treatment of any underlying disease.[16,17]

Symptom Control

C1-INH-AAE symptom management is based on existing knowledge regarding effective therapies for HAE. Symptomatic treatment is achieved by regulating bradykinin activity using therapies found to be effective in HAE.

At baseline, avoidance of triggers reported to exacerbate bradykinin-mediated angioedema is recommended (social stressors, trauma, exogenous estrogens, tamoxifen, ACEIs). As C1-INH-AAE can present with laryngeal edema,[60–62] an emergency care plan should be in place, and a written treatment plan for emergency care should be provided.[17] Patients should have appropriate access to kallikrein-bradykinin–targeted therapies as part of their acute treatment and prophylaxis plans.

Acute Treatment

Acute treatment aims to reduce the severity and duration of each acute attack.[63] It was noted at the 2014 bradykinin-mediated angioedema expert consensus meeting that C1-INH concentrate can be effective in treating acute attacks. However, acute treatment of C1-INH-AAE differs from HAE in that some cases of C1-INH-AAE may

Table 1
Complement level patterns for hereditary and acquired C1 esterase inhibitor deficiencies

Diagnosis	C1-INH	C1-INH Function	C4	C1q	Anti-C1-INH
HAE with C1-INH deficiency	Low	Low	Low	Normal	Absent
HAE type II	Normal	Low	Low	Normal	Absent
AAE type I	Low	Low	Low	Low	Absent
AAE type II	Low/normal	Low	Low	Low	Present

be resistant to treatment with C1-INH concentrate. Higher doses of C1-INH concentrate are often required to achieve a therapeutic response, especially in patients with anti-C1-INH autoantibodies.[21]

Published literature has reported the successful use of icatibant, a bradykinin B2 receptor antagonist, and ecallantide, a kallikrein inhibitor, in treating acute AAE attacks.[64,65] In an observational study, icatibant was effective at treating 47 of 48 attacks in 8 patients with AAE.[65] Icatibant was also able to effectively treat facial and laryngeal AAE attacks resistant to treatment with C1-INH concentrate.[57] Ecallantide was able to effectively treat facial attacks in patients who did not respond or only partially responded to C1-INH concentrate.[57,64] The fact that a bradykinin B2 receptor antagonist is able to treat acute attacks resistant to C1-INH concentrate highlights the importance of bradykinin binding to the bradykinin B2 receptor as a key step in symptom development.

Prophylaxis

Prophylactic therapy aims to prevent or reduce the frequency and severity of acute attacks (long-term prophylaxis) or prevent attacks during planned exposure to known attack triggers such as surgical procedures (short-term prophylaxis).[63]

Short-term Prophylaxis

C1-INH concentrate was recommended for short-term prophylaxis at the 2014 bradykinin-mediated angioedema expert consensus meeting based on unpublished cases discussed at this meeting.[21] In a case series of 10 patients with C1-INH-AAE, 5 patients received androgen therapy, 1 patient received C1-INH replacement, and 4 patients received no prophylaxis preoperatively. Significant perioperative airway complications or angioedema episodes were not reported in these patients.[66]

Long-term Prophylaxis

C1-INH concentrate can also be used for long-term prophylaxis. C1-INH concentrate must be dosed at a minimum of twice a week, and long-term prophylaxis with C1-INH concentrate is often considered only for select patients who have 2 or more severe attacks per week.[57] If long-term prophylaxis is necessary, self-intravenous administration is possible and can help improve patients' quality of life.[58]

Tranexamic acid has been used successfully for prophylactic therapy.[7,57,58,67–69] However, tranexamic acid has potential adverse effects, and the risk for thromboembolism is particularly concerning for AAE patients with underlying malignancies.[17]

Androgens are an effective treatment option for C1-INH-AAE.[58] Long-term use of androgens must be accompanied by routine monitoring of transaminases, lipids, blood pressure, weight, menstrual irregularities, and liver ultrasonography.[58] Given this adverse side-effect profile and comparative lack of efficacy in C1-INH-AAE, the other previously mentioned therapeutic options are generally preferred over androgens, but patient preference is strongly considered.

Fresh frozen plasma (FFP) has not been investigated for the treatment of C1-INH-AAE.[21] In HAE, concerns have been raised regarding the potential for FFP to cause acute worsening of symptoms, although a subsequent publication of 23 case reports (combined original case series and literature review) did not identify any exacerbation of attacks with FFP.[70] For now, the authors recommend avoiding FFP for C1-INH-AAE patients until it has been investigated specifically in the C1-INH-AAE population.

Treatment of Acquired Angioedema due to C1-INH Deficiency and Underlying Systemic Conditions

Successful control of associated conditions can lead to partial or complete remission of symptoms and reversal of complement abnormalities.

Rituximab has been used successfully to treat C1-INH-AAE. In many cases, rituximab can induce long-lasting remission of angioedema with normalization of C1-INH. Rituximab can be effective in cases that were refractory to corticosteroid and/or cyclophosphamide therapies (**Table 2**). The presence or absence of lymphoproliferative disease, and the presence or absence of anti-C1-INH autoantibody, does not appear to be consistently associated with the degree of response to rituximab (see **Table 2**).

Chemotherapy regimens used to treat underlying malignant lymphoproliferative disease have been associated with C1-INH-AAE remission in 9 cases.[76–81]

PROGNOSIS

Once a diagnosis of C1-INH-AAE has been made, subsequent evaluation for systemic underlying medical conditions, such as lymphoproliferative and/or autoimmune disorders, is warranted.[38] The prevalence of lymphoproliferative disease in C1-INH-AAE has been reported to be higher than 70%.[10]

Even if an initial evaluation does not reveal a clear diagnosis of underlying conditions, routine monitoring is warranted. Patients without lymphoproliferative disease at time of C1-INH-AAE diagnosis can subsequently develop lymphoproliferative disease.[7,32,82] In addition, patients with C1-INH-AAE are at higher risk of developing NHL compared with the general population.[67,80,81]

Resolution of C1-INH-AAE appears to be associated with successful treatment of underlying lymphoproliferative and/or autoimmune disease. Reported cases of C1-INH-AAE treated with rituximab or chemotherapy have largely resulted in complete, or at least partial, remission (see **Table 2**).

CURRENT CONTROVERSIES
Pathophysiology

As mentioned under the Pathophysiology section, C1-INH-AAE has historically been classified into type I (without anti-C1-INH autoantibody) and type II (with anti-C1-INH autoantibody). However, published reports show that although C1-INH-AAE can be a clinical manifestation of LPD and systemic autoimmunity,[23–31] LPD can lead to both C1-INH-AAE with and without anti-C1-INH autoantibodies, and systemic autoimmunity can lead to C1-INH-AAE in the absence of anti-C1-INH autoantibodies.[10,32–37] It remains to be determined whether C1-INH-AAE cases represent a clinical spectrum of one pathophysiologic process, or if these C1-INH-AAE cases represent distinct entities. To answer this question, detailed studies investigating the disease processes leading to C1-INH-AAE are needed.

C1 Esterase Inhibitor Replacement Therapy

C1-INH-AAE cases can be relatively resistant to C1-INH replacement (ie, higher doses of C1-INH replacement are often required to achieve a therapeutic response).[21] It has been proposed that long-term prophylaxis may lead to C1-INH resistance.[57] The presence of anti-C1-INH autoantibodies tends to be associated with C1-INH resistance.[21]

It remains to be definitively determined if the use of C1-INH replacement for long-term prophylaxis does in fact lead to C1-INH resistance. This question is important

Table 2
Acquired angioedema due to C1-INH deficiency treated with rituximab: baseline characteristics of patients and response to therapy

Author	Age	G	Location	Anti-c1-INH	Underlying Condition	RTX	Symptom Remission	C4	C1-INH	C1-INHf	Anti-C1-INH	Other Immunosuppressive Therapy
Lam et al,[71] 2012	80	F	Abdomen	NR	Splenic marginal zone lymphoma	1	Complete	—	N	—	—	—
Ziakas et al,[72] 2004	67	M	Abdomen	Yes	Clonal B-cell 2% infiltration of bone marrow	1	Partial	—	—	—	—	1
Levi et al,[73] 2006	45	F	NR	Yes (IgG)	None	1	Complete	N	N	—	—	2
Levi et al,[73] 2006	70	F	NR	No	Stage IV indolent follicular B-cell lymphoma	1	Complete	I	I	—	—	—
Levi et al,[73] 2006	68	M	NR	No	None	1	Complete	N	N	—	—	2
Hassan et al,[74] 2011	84	F	Extremities face	Yes (IgM)	MGUS (IgM)	1	Partial	—	—	—	D	—
Branellec et al,[60] 2012	54	F	Abdomen extremities genitalia	Yes (IgM)	None	2	Partial	—	N	I	D	3
Branellec et al,[60] 2012	79	M	Extremities genitalia	Yes (Igm)	MZL	2	Complete	—	N	I	D	4
Branellec et al,[60] 2012	61	M	Face	Yes (IgA)	MGUS (IgA)	1[a]	Ineffective	—	U	—	—	3
Branellec et al,[60] 2012	51	F	Abdomen	Yes (IgG)	MGUS (IgG)	1	Complete	—	U	U	I	3
Branellec et al,[60] 2012	82	F	Larynx	Yes (IgM)	None	1	Partial	—	U	—	U	—

(continued on next page)

Table 2
(continued)

Author	Age	G	Location	Anti-c1-INH	Underlying Condition	RTX	Symptom Remission	C4	C1-INH	C1-INHf	Anti-C1-INH	Other Immunosuppressive Therapy
Branellec et al,[60] 2012	80	F	Face	Yes (IgM)	MGUS (IgG)	1[b]	Partial	—	U	—	—	—
Branellec et al,[60] 2012	75	F	Face	No	MZL	2	Partial	—	I	—	—	3
Bygum & Vestergaard,[7] 2013	46	M	NR	No	SLL	NR	Partial	—	—	—	—	—
Bygum & Vestergaard,[7] 2013	69	M	NR	Yes (IgM)	Monoclonal B-cell lymphocytosis	1	Deceased	—	—	—	—	—
Kaur et al,[62] 2014	51	M	Larynx	NR	Monoclonal B-cell lymphocytosis	1	Complete	—	—	—	—	—
Dreyfus et al,[61] 2014	41	F	Larynx abdomen	Yes (IgG)	Myasthenia gravis, antiphospholipid syndrome	1	Complete	—	—	—	N	—
Sanchez-Cano et al,[75] 2008	66	F	NR	Yes (IgM)	Sjogren Syndrome	2	Complete	—	—	—	D	—

Abbreviations: 1, monthly cyclophosphamide lead to remission but was stopped due to pneumocystis jirovecii pneumonia; 2, prednisolone (50 mg/d) in combination with cyclophosphamide (150 mg/d) ineffective; 3, corticosteroids ineffective; 4, 6 cycles of cyclophosphamide starting with third dose of RTX; Age, age in years; C1-INHF, c1 inhibitor esterase function; D, decreased; G, gender; I, increased; NR, not reported; Partial, decrease in severity and/or frequency of angioedema attacks; R, number of rituximab cycles (1 cycle is 375 mg/m^2/wk for 4 weeks); RTX, Rituximab; U, unchanged.

[a] Followed by 1-g infusion 1 year later.

[b] Followed by four 1-g infusions over the following 3 years.

because it affects the decision to place patients on long-term prophylaxis with C1-INH concentrate.

It also remains to be established whether the presence of anti-C1-INH autoantibodies do indeed predict C1-INH resistance. Recommended starting doses of C1-INH concentrate may need to be higher for C1-INH-AAE with anti-C1-INH autoantibodies.

Rituximab Therapy

A diagnosis of C1-INH-AAE can precede a diagnosis of lymphoproliferative disease[7,32,82] and confers an increased risk for developing NHL.[67,80,81] An isolated case suggests that rituximab therapy for C1-INH-AAE without any underlying conditions and without detectable anti-C1-INH autoantibody can be successful at achieving angioedema symptom remission.[73] Whether rituximab therapy for C1-INH-AAE without any known underlying conditions may help prevent future development of lymphoproliferative and autoimmune disease is unknown.

REFERENCES

1. Caldwell JR, Ruddy S, Schur PH, et al. Acquired C1 inhibitor deficiency in lymphosarcoma. Clin Immunol Immunopathol 1972;1(1):39–52.
2. Cicardi M. Acquired C1 inhibitor deficiency: clinical manifestations, epidemiology, pathogenesis, and diagnosis - UpToDate. Available at: https://www.uptodate.com/contents/acquired-c1-inhibitor-deficiency-clinical-manifestations-epidemiology-pathogenesis-and-diagnosis?source=search_result&search=acquiredangioedema&selectedTitle=1~32. Accessed December 4, 2016.
3. Mansi M, Zanichelli A, Coerezza A, et al. Presentation, diagnosis and treatment of angioedema without wheals: a retrospective analysis of a cohort of 1058 patients. J Intern Med 2015;277(5):585–93.
4. Zingale LC, Beltrami L, Zanichelli A, et al. Angioedema without urticaria: a large clinical survey. CMAJ 2006;175(9):1065–70.
5. Breitbart SI, Bielory L. Acquired angioedema: autoantibody associations and C1q utility as a diagnostic tool. Allergy Asthma Proc 2010;31(5):428–34.
6. Jolles S, Williams P, Carne E, et al. A UK national audit of hereditary and acquired angioedema. Clin Exp Immunol 2014;175(1):59–67.
7. Bygum A, Vestergaard H. Acquired angioedema–occurrence, clinical features and associated disorders in a Danish nationwide patient cohort. Int Arch Allergy Immunol 2013;162(2):149–55.
8. Cicardi M, Johnston DT. Hereditary and acquired complement component 1 esterase inhibitor deficiency: a review for the hematologist. Acta Haematol 2012;127(4):208–20.
9. Gobert D, Paule R, Ponard D, et al. A nationwide study of acquired C1-inhibitor deficiency in France. Medicine (Baltimore) 2016;95(33):e4363.
10. Cicardi M, Zanichelli A. The acquired deficiency of C1-inhibitor: lymphoproliferation and angioedema. Curr Mol Med 2010;10(4):354–60.
11. Agostoni A, Aygören-Pürsün E, Binkley KE, et al. Hereditary and acquired angioedema: problems and progress: proceedings of the third C1 esterase inhibitor deficiency workshop and beyond. J Allergy Clin Immunol 2004;114(3):S51–131.
12. Lang DM, Aberer W, Bernstein JA, et al. International consensus on hereditary and acquired angioedema. Ann Allergy Asthma Immunol 2012;109(6):395–402.
13. Bouillet-Claveyrolas L, Ponard D, Drouet C, et al. Clinical and biological distinctions between type I and type II acquired angioedema. Am J Med 2003;115(5):420–1.

14. Dobson G, Edgar D, Trinder J. Angioedema of the tongue due to acquired C1 esterase inhibitor deficiency. Anaesth Intensive Care 2003;31(1):99–102. Available at: http://www.ncbi.nlm.nih.gov/pubmed/12635405. Accessed December 3, 2016.

15. Eck SL, Morse JH, Janssen DA, et al. Angioedema presenting as chronic gastrointestinal symptoms. Am J Gastroenterol 1993;88(3):436–9. Available at: http://www.ncbi.nlm.nih.gov/pubmed/8438855. Accessed December 3, 2016.

16. Bork K. An evidence based therapeutic approach to hereditary and acquired angioedema. Curr Opin Allergy Clin Immunol 2014;14(4):354–62.

17. Wu MA, Castelli R. The Janus faces of acquired angioedema: C1-inhibitor deficiency, lymphoproliferation and autoimmunity. Clin Chem Lab Med 2016;54(2):207–14.

18. Jacobsen S. Separation of 2 different substrates for plasma kinin-forming enzymes. Nature 1966;210(5031):98–9. Available at: http://www.ncbi.nlm.nih.gov/pubmed/4163182. Accessed November 25, 2016.

19. Campbell DJ. The kallikrein-kinin system in humans. Clin Exp Pharmacol Physiol 2001;28(12):1060–5. Available at: http://www.ncbi.nlm.nih.gov/pubmed/11903316. Accessed November 25, 2016.

20. Zeerleder S, Levi M. Hereditary and acquired C1-inhibitor-dependent angioedema: from pathophysiology to treatment. Ann Med 2016;48(4):256–67.

21. Craig TJ, Bernstein JA, Farkas H, et al. Diagnosis and treatment of bradykinin-mediated angioedema: outcomes from an angioedema expert consensus meeting. Int Arch Allergy Immunol 2014;165(2):119–27.

22. Alsenz J, Bork K, Loos M. Autoantibody-mediated acquired deficiency of C1 inhibitor. N Engl J Med 1987;316(22):1360–6.

23. Schreiber AD, Zweiman B, Atkins P, et al. Acquired angioedema with lymphoproliferative disorder: association of C1 inhibitor deficiency with cellular abnormality. Blood 1976;48(4):567–80. Available at: http://www.ncbi.nlm.nih.gov/pubmed/1085645. Accessed November 25, 2016.

24. Mathur R, Toghill PJ, Johnston ID. Acquired C1 inhibitor deficiency with lymphoma causing recurrent angioedema. Postgrad Med J 1993;69(814):646–8. Available at: http://www.ncbi.nlm.nih.gov/pubmed/8234113. Accessed November 25, 2016.

25. Hauptmann G, Mayer S, Lang JM, et al. Treatment of acquired C1-inhibitor deficiency with danazol. Ann Intern Med 1977;87(5):577–8. Available at: http://www.ncbi.nlm.nih.gov/pubmed/921088. Accessed November 25, 2016.

26. Hauptmann G, Lang JM, North ML, et al. Acquired c1-inhibitor deficiencies in lymphoproliferative diseases with serum immunoglobulin abnormalities. A study of three cases. Blut 1976;32(3):195–206. Available at: http://www.ncbi.nlm.nih.gov/pubmed/946413. Accessed November 25, 2016.

27. Day NK, Winfield JB, Gee T, et al. Evidence for immune complexes involving anti-lymphocyte antibodies associated with hypocomplementaemia in chronic lymphocytic leukaemia (CLL). Clin Exp Immunol 1976;26(2):189–95. Available at: http://www.ncbi.nlm.nih.gov/pubmed/136325. Accessed November 25, 2016.

28. Cohen SH, Koethe SM. Danazol and C1 esterase inhibitor deficiency. Ann Intern Med 1978;88(3):429. Available at: http://www.ncbi.nlm.nih.gov/pubmed/629510. Accessed November 25, 2016.

29. Hauptmann G, Petitjean F, Lang JM, et al. Acquired C1 inhibitor deficiency in a case of lymphosarcoma of the spleen. Reversal of complement abnormalities after splenectomy. Clin Exp Immunol 1979;37(3):523–31. Available at: http://www.pubmedcentral.nih.gov/articlerender.fcgi?artid=1537769&tool=pmcentrez&rendertype=abstract.

30. Geha RS, Quinti I, Austen KF, et al. Acquired C1-inhibitor deficiency associated with antiidiotypic antibody to monoclonal immunoglobulins. N Engl J Med 1985;312(9):534–40.
31. Jackson J, Sim R, Whelan A, et al. An IgG autoantibody which inactivates C1-inhibitor. Nature 1986;320:264–5.
32. Cicardi M, Beretta A, Colombo M, et al. Relevance of lymphoproliferative disorders and of anti-C1 inhibitor autoantibodies in acquired angio-oedema. Clin Exp Immunol 1996;106(3):475–80.
33. Cacoub P, Frémeaux-Bacchi V, De Lacroix I, et al. A new type of acquired C1 inhibitor deficiency associated with systemic lupus erythematosus. Arthritis Rheum 2001;44(8):1836–40.
34. Jazwinska EC, Gatenby PA, Dunckley H, et al. C1 inhibitor functional deficiency in systemic lupus erythematosus (SLE). Clin Exp Immunol 1993;92:268–73.
35. Nakamura S, Yoshinari M, Saku Y, et al. Acquired C 1 inhibitor deficiency associated with systemic lupus erythematosus affecting the central nervous system. Ann Rheum Dis 1991;50(10):713–6. Available at: http://ard.bmj.com/content/50/10/713.short.
36. Nettis E, Colanardi MC, Loria MP, et al. Acquired C1-inhibitor deficiency in a patient with systemic lupus erythematosus: a case report and review of the literature. Eur J Clin Invest 2005;35(12):781–4.
37. Sugisaki K, Itoh K, Tamaru JI. Acquired C1-esterase inhibitor deficiency and positive lupus anticoagulant accompanied by splenic marginal zone B-cell lymphoma. Clin Exp Rheumatol 2007;25(4):627–9.
38. Farkas H, Veszeli N, Kajdácsi E, et al. "Nuts and bolts" of laboratory evaluation of angioedema. Clin Rev Allergy Immunol 2016;51:1–12.
39. Fenny N, Grammer LC. Idiopathic anaphylaxis. Immunol Allergy Clin North Am 2015;35(2):349–62.
40. Bernstein JA, Lang DM, Khan DA, et al. The diagnosis and management of acute and chronic urticaria: 2014 update. J Allergy Clin Immunol 2014;133(5):1270–7.e66.
41. González-de-Olano D, Matito A, Orfao A, et al. Advances in the understanding and clinical management of mastocytosis and clonal mast cell activation syndromes. F1000Research 2016;5:2666.
42. Lee S, Hess EP, Lohse C, et al. Trends, characteristics, and incidence of anaphylaxis in 2001-2010: a population-based study. J Allergy Clin Immunol 2016;139(1):182–8.e2.
43. Golden DBK, Moffitt J, Nicklas RA, et al. Stinging insect hypersensitivity: a practice parameter update 2011. J Allergy Clin Immunol 2011;127(4):852–4.e23.
44. Tam JS. Cutaneous manifestation of food allergy. Immunol Allergy Clin North Am 2017;37(1):217–31.
45. Larson AM. Palliative care for patients with end-stage liver disease. Curr Gastroenterol Rep 2015;17(5):18.
46. Alpert CM, Smith MA, Hummel SL, et al. Symptom burden in heart failure: assessment, impact on outcomes, and management. Heart Fail Rev 2016;22:1–15.
47. Rheault M, Gbadegesin R. The genetics of nephrotic syndrome. J Pediatr Genet 2015;5(1):015–24.
48. Khoury P, Herold J, Alpaugh A, et al. Episodic angioedema with eosinophilia (Gleich syndrome) is a multilineage cell cycling disorder. Haematologica 2015;100(3):300–7.
49. Shikino K, Hirose Y, Nakagawa S, et al. Non-episodic angioedema associated with eosinophilia. BMJ Case Rep 2016;2016.

50. Lucchini G, Willasch AM, Daniel J, et al. Epidemiology, risk factors, and prognosis of capillary leak syndrome in pediatric recipients of stem cell transplants: a retrospective single-center cohort study. Pediatr Transplant 2016;20(8):1132–6.

51. Singh Bakshi S. Melkersson-Rosenthal syndrome. J Allergy Clin Immunol Pract 2017;5(2):471–2.

52. Kirkpatrick CH. A mechanism for urticaria/angioedema in patients with thyroid disease. J Allergy Clin Immunol 2012;130(4):988–90.

53. Karagol HIE, Yilmaz O, Topal E, et al. Association between thyroid autoimmunity and recurrent angioedema in children. Allergy Asthma Proc 2015;36(6):468–72.

54. Saff RR, Banerji A. Management of patients with nonaspirin-exacerbated respiratory disease aspirin hypersensitivity reactions. Allergy Asthma Proc 2015;36(1): 34–9.

55. Kaplan AP. Bradykinin-mediated diseases. Chem Immunol Allergy 2014;100: 140–7.

56. Baram M, Kommuri A, Sellers SA, et al. ACE inhibitor–induced angioedema. J Allergy Clin Immunol Pract 2013;1:442–5.

57. Cicardi M, Zanichelli A. Acquired angioedema. Allergy Asthma Clin Immunol 2010;6(1):14.

58. Cicardi M, Aberer W, Banerji A, et al. Classification, diagnosis, and approach to treatment for angioedema: consensus report from the Hereditary Angioedema International Working Group. Allergy 2014;69(5):602–16.

59. Oltvai ZN, Wong EC, Atkinson JP, et al. C1 inhibitor deficiency: molecular and immunologic basis of hereditary and acquired angioedema. Lab Investig A J Tech Methods Pathol 2016;65(4):381–8.

60. Branellec A, Bouillet L, Javaud N, et al. Acquired C1-inhibitor deficiency: 7 patients treated with rituximab. J Clin Immunol 2012;32(5):936–41.

61. Dreyfus DH, Na CR, Randolph CC, et al. Successful rituximab B lymphocyte depletion therapy for angioedema due to acquired C1 inhibitor protein deficiency: association with reduced C1 inhibitor protein autoantibody titers. Isr Med Assoc J 2014;16(5):315–6. Available at: http://www.ncbi.nlm.nih.gov/ pubmed/24979840. Accessed November 28, 2016.

62. Kaur R, Williams AA, Swift CB, et al. Rituximab therapy in a patient with low grade B-cell lymphoproliferative disease and concomitant acquired angioedema. J Asthma Allergy 2014;7:165–7.

63. Bowen T, Cicardi M, Farkas H, et al. 2010 International consensus algorithm for the diagnosis, therapy and management of hereditary angioedema. Allergy. Asthma Clin Immunol 2010;6(1):24.

64. Patel NS, Fung SM, Zanichelli A, et al. Ecallantide for treatment of acute attacks of acquired C1 esterase inhibitor deficiency. Allergy Asthma Proc 2013;34(1):72–7.

65. Zanichelli A, Bova M, Coerezza A, et al. Icatibant treatment for acquired C1-inhibitor deficiency: a real-world observational study. Allergy 2012;67(8):1074–7.

66. MacBeth LS, Volcheck GW, Sprung J, et al. Perioperative course in patients with hereditary or acquired angioedema. J Clin Anesth 2016;34:385–91.

67. Cugno M, Cicardi M, Agostoni A. Activation of the contact system and fibrinolysis in autoimmune acquired angioedema: a rationale for prophylactic use of tranexamic acid. J Allergy Clin Immunol 1994;93(5):870–6. Available at: http://www.ncbi. nlm.nih.gov/pubmed/8182230. Accessed November 27, 2016.

68. Du-Thanh A, Raison-Peyron N, Drouet C, et al. Efficacy of tranexamic acid in sporadic idiopathic bradykinin angioedema. Allergy 2009;65(6):793–5.

69. Cicardi M, Bergamaschini L, Zingale LC, et al. Idiopathic nonhistaminergic angioedema. Am J Med 1999;106(6):650–4. Available at: http://www.ncbi.nlm.nih.gov/pubmed/10378623. Accessed November 27, 2016.
70. Prematta M, Gibbs JG, Pratt EL, et al. Fresh frozen plasma for the treatment of hereditary angioedema. Ann Allergy Asthma Immunol 2007;98(4):383–8.
71. Lam DH, Levy NB, Nickerson JM, et al. Acquired angioedema and marginal zone lymphoma. J Clin Oncol 2012;30(16):e151–3.
72. Ziakas PD, Giannouli S, Psimenou E, et al. Acquired angioedema: a new target for rituximab? Haematologica 2004;89(8):ELT13. Available at: http://www.ncbi.nlm.nih.gov/pubmed/15339702. Accessed November 27, 2016.
73. Levi M, Hack CE, van Oers MH. Rituximab-induced elimination of acquired angioedema due to C1-inhibitor deficiency. Am J Med 2006;119(8):e3–5.
74. Hassan A, Amarger S, Tridon A, et al. Acquired angioedema responding to rituximab. Acta Derm Venereol 2011;91(6):733–4.
75. Sanchez-Cano D, Callejas-Rubio J, Lara-Jimenez M, et al. Successful use of rituximab in acquired C1 inhibitor deficiency secondary to Sjogren's syndrome. Lupus 2008;17(3):228–9.
76. Rossi D, Gaidano G. Anaplastic large cell lymphoma and acquired angioedema: a novel association? Ann Ital Med Int 2002;17(3):143–5. Available at: http://www.ncbi.nlm.nih.gov/pubmed/12402660. Accessed November 29, 2016.
77. Healy C, Abuzakouk M, Feighery C, et al. Acquired angioedema in non-Hodgkin's lymphoma. Oral Surg Oral Med Oral Pathol Oral Radiol Endod 2007;103(5):e29–32.
78. Guilarte M, Luengo O, Nogueiras C, et al. Acquired angioedema associated with hereditary angioedema due to C1 inhibitor deficiency. J Investig Allergol Clin Immunol 2008;18(2):126–30. Available at: http://www.ncbi.nlm.nih.gov/pubmed/18447143. Accessed November 29, 2016.
79. Jung M, Rice L. Unusual autoimmune nonhematologic complications in chronic lymphocytic leukemia. Clin Lymphoma Myeloma Leuk 2011;11(Suppl 1):S10–3.
80. Castelli R, Deliliers DL, Zingale LC, et al. Lymphoproliferative disease and acquired C1 inhibitor deficiency. Haematologica 2007;92(5):716–8. Available at: http://www.ncbi.nlm.nih.gov/pubmed/17488706. Accessed November 29, 2016.
81. Castelli R, Zanichelli A, Cicardi M, et al. Acquired C1-inhibitor deficiency and lymphoproliferative disorders: a tight relationship. Crit Rev Oncol Hematol 2013;87(3):323–32.
82. Cicardi M, Zingale LC, Pappalardo E, et al. Autoantibodies and lymphoproliferative diseases in acquired C1-inhibitor deficiencies. Medicine (Baltimore) 2003;82(4):274–81.

Pathogenesis of Hereditary Angioedema

The Role of the Bradykinin-Forming Cascade

Allen P. Kaplan, MD[a],*, Kusumam Joseph, PhD[b]

KEYWORDS

- Factor XII • Prekallikrein • Kininogen • Bradykinin • Angioedema

KEY POINTS

- Attacks of swelling in types I and II hereditary angioedema (HAE) are due to overproduction of bradykinin.
- HAE types I and II are caused by mutations in the gene encoding C1 inhibitor (C1-INH) so that patients are functionally deficient.
- C1-INH blocks plasma kallikrein and the 2 molecular forms of activated factor XII, enzymes requisite for bradykinin formation and stabilizes the prekallikrein-high molecular kininogen complex.
- Therapies for types I and II HAE include C1-INH replacement, inhibition of the enzyme kallikrein, and blockade at the bradykinin B-2 receptor.

INTRODUCTION

Hereditary angioedema (HAE) represents a prototypic disorder in which episodic swelling, that is, angioedema, is dependent on the generation of bradykinin. In contrast with the ingestion of inhibitors of angiotensin-converting enzyme, which cause accumulation of bradykinin owing to impaired degradation, all forms of HAE in which the pathogenesis is understood, seem to be due to overproduction of bradykinin. The first described entity is C1 inhibitor (C1-INH) deficiency,[1] in which absent or dysfunctional C1-INH lessens inhibition of key enzymes required for bradykinin formation. Decades later, a novel form of HAE was described in which C1-INH levels are normal.[2,3] About one-third of the latter cases (but varies greatly worldwide) have a mutation in factor XII,[4,5] which leads to an increased rate of factor XII activation and augmented bradykinin formation. There is no genetic abnormality or mechanistic

Disclosure: Research grant funding from CSL Behring and Shire Pharmaceuticals.
[a] Department of Medicine, Medical University of South Carolina, 171 Ashley Avenue, Charleston, SC 29425, USA; [b] Department of Biochemistry and Molecular Biology, Medical University of South Carolina, 173 Ashley Avenue, Charleston, SC 29425, USA
* Corresponding author. 17 Logan Street, Charleston, SC 29401.
E-mail address: Kaplana@musc.edu

rationale involving the remaining two-thirds of subjects, although indirect evidence, for example, response to agents that are effective in other types of HAE, suggest that this entity also depends on bradykinin production. Those lacking any defined mutation are distinguished from idiopathic angioedema by a clear family history of recurrent angioedema. This review addresses the major pathophysiologic mechanisms operative in HAE of each type.

THE ROLE OF C1 INHIBITOR IN COMPLEMENT ACTIVATION

C1-INH was named because it inhibited the activated form of the first component of complement.[6] More specifically, it inhibits activated C1r and activated C1s of the C1 complex. The formula of C1 is actually $C1q (C1r)_2 (C1s)_2$.[7] C1q is the key structure to which immune complexes bind and consists of 6 globular heads and a lengthy collagen-like tail. Two molecules each of C1r and C1s bind to the collagen tail in calcium-dependent reactions. Thus, chelation of calcium by EDTA disrupts C1 and activation cannot proceed. When immune complexes bind to C1, C1r is initially activated by a conformational change (C1r*) and the 2 C1r* digest each other to yield C1r̄, which is cleaved and fully active.[8] C1r̄ digests C1s to C1s̄ and C1 and C1s digests its 2 substrates, C4 and C2 (**Fig. 1**) to yield C4a (anaphylatoxin) and C4b and C2a and C2b, respectively. The labile component of the C1 complex is clearly C1r because, when purified, it autoactivates and autodigests to C1r̄ (**Fig. 2**).[8] When the entire C1 complex is purified, it too autoactivates, but much more slowly than purified C1r and the autoactivation phenomenon is inhibited by the C1-INH; that is, the complex is stabilized.[9] When an immune complex activates C1, each C1r̄ and each C1s̄ binds irreversibly to C1-INH to yield $(C1\bar{r})_2 - (C1\text{-INH})_2$ and $(C1\bar{s})_2 (C1\text{-INH})_2$ so that 4 C1-INH molecules are "used up."

When C1-INH is absent or dysfunctional, as is the case for types I and II HAE, respectively, the stabilization of C1 is lessened such that C1 is partially activated and C4, the preferred substrate of C1s̄ is depleted. C4 levels are low in 95% of patients[10]; thus, it is a good (but not perfect) biomarker for the likelihood of types I or II HAE in patients with recurrent angioedema. When suspected, blood levels of C1-INH are typically drawn at the same time and quantitated both as a protein and

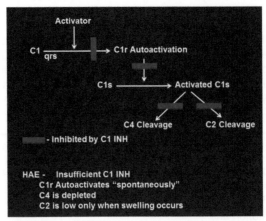

Fig. 1. The activation mechanism for the first component of complement leading to diminished levels of C4 and C2 in patients with hereditary angioedema (HAE). C1-INH, C1 inhibitor.

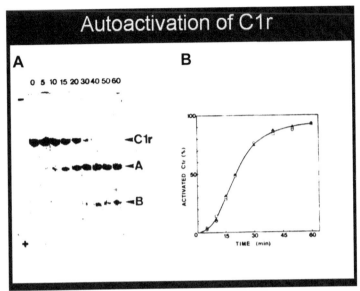

Fig. 2. Autoactivation of purified C1r. A 1-hour time course (*left*) demonstrating cleavage of C1r within a disulfide bridge as assessed by reduced SDS gel electrophoresis to yield as (*A*) heavy chain and (*B*) light chain. The time course of activity (ie, activated C1r) is shown on the right. (*From* Arlaud GJ, Villiers CL, Chesne S, et al. Purified proenzyme C1r. Some characteristics of its activation and subsequent proteolytic cleavage. Biochimica et Biophysica Acta 1980;616:119.)

functional level. In type I patients (85% of C1-INH deficiency), both are low, whereas type II patients (15% of C1-INH deficiency) have a normal or even elevated protein level, but a functional level that is just as low as type I patients. In general, the difference is in the nature of the mutation. Type I subjects tend to have deletions, insertions, or duplications that disrupt transcription and the partial polypeptide is degraded or not secreted. Type II patients usually have an amino acid substitution that affects function, although the protein is secreted normally. In either case, the mutation typically affects only 1 gene, so the disorder transmits as an autosomal-dominant change. Homozygous mutations are very rare. Because there is 1 unaffected gene, one might expect a blood level of 50% C1-INH in all patients. However, functional levels typically range from a few percent to about 35%, a range in which attacks of angioedema are seen. It seems that transcription of the normal gene is inhibited (transinhibition)[11] at the messenger RNA level. In addition, functional C1-INH will be further depleted by binding to enzymes whose activity it controls.[12]

BRADYKININ IS THE MEDIATOR OF SWELLING IN HEREDITARY ANGIOEDEMA TYPES I AND II

Although patients have a low C4 level at baseline, the C2 level is normal. However, when attacks of angioedema occur, C4 levels decrease further and C2 is depleted,[13] indicating that there is further activation of C1, apparently in the absence of immune complexes. Donaldson and coworkers[14] suspected that a vasoactive peptide might be liberated from complement, that is, C2 in particular, to cause angioedema and called the product C2 kinin. They reported that when C2 is activated to C2a and C2b, the C2a is further digested by plasmin to release the kinin.[14] A number of observations seemed to corroborate this view. For example, the intradermal injection of activated C1 (or C1s) led to a wheal, that is, an increase in vascular permeability, that was lessened in the absence of C2.[15] In addition, the smooth muscle contractile activity of plasmin-derived C2 kinin was destroyed by digestion with trypsin, which has no effect on bradykinin.[14] Nevertheless, after decades passed, no such peptide was identified. Curd and colleagues[16] demonstrated that the concentration of plasma kallikrein, a bradykinin-forming enzyme, in induced blisters of HAE patients (C1-INH deficiency) was greater than observed in normal controls. This corroborated earlier evidence that C1-INH inhibits plasma kallikrein[17] so that increased activity is observed with C1-INH deficiency, but did not address activation of the cascade in patients' plasma or the C2 kinin controversy. In 1983, Fields and colleagues[18] reported that activation of C1, C4, and C2 followed by plasmin digestion of failed to produce any kinin based on contractile activity. Further, they noted that plasma of HAE patients incubated at 37°C in the absence of an activator of the bradykinin-forming cascade, produced bradykinin seemingly spontaneously with progressively increasing levels during the time course. They concluded that bradykinin and not C2 kinin is the mediator of the swelling. It is difficult, in retrospect, to explain the findings that suggested a "C2 kinin," but one issue relates to the assay used for contractile activity. We found the estrus rat uterus, used originally, to have an unstable baseline and that contractions could be induced simply by disturbing the suspension bath with buffer. A guinea pig ilium strip was stable and reproducible results were obtained. Further, injecting any substance into human skin (eg, C1) will activate the bradykinin cascade, although a lesser response with C2 deficiency cannot be explained. The inability to generate a kininlike molecule from C2 was confirmed soon thereafter,[19] but additional support for bradykinin as the mediator of HAE took much longer.

Shoemaker and colleagues[20] reported that the only kinin that could be generated in HAE plasma was bradykinin and that plasma deficient in C2 behaved normally, in contradistinction to earlier reports. Thus, the results reported by Fields and colleagues[20] were confirmed, albeit with a differing methodology. Deficient plasma was used instead of purified C2 and bradykinin was measured by radioimmunoassay (developed in the ensuing decade) rather than bioassay. Next, a family was described in which C1-INH seemed deficient based on inhibition of C1 but had normal function as an inhibitor of bradykinin-forming enzymes. The result was that there was no angioedema in any family member,[21] again demonstrating that abnormal complement activation is not the answer. Nussberger and colleagues[22] measured bradykinin levels in HAE patients during acute attacks of angioedema and demonstrated elevated levels at the site of swelling demonstrating bradykinin as the in vivo mediator, which also suggested that its initial production is a localized process. A rat model of C1-INH deficiency led to an increase in vascular permeability that could be reversed by deleting the B2 bradykinin receptor.[23] The final observation was that icatibant, which binds to the bradykinin B2 receptor and inhibits bradykinin reactivity rapidly, reverses attacks of angioedema in HAE patients[24] and a plasma kallikrein inhibitor has similar efficacy.[25]

Recently, there has been consideration that des-arg^9-bradykinin, a bradykinin metabolite that retains the ability to increase vascular permeability could contribute to the angioedema of HAE types I and II. Des-arg^9-bradykinin is generated by digestion of bradykinin by carboxypeptidase N in plasma[26] and carboxypeptidase M on the surface of vascular endothelial cells.[27] It binds to B1 receptors rather than B2 receptors and B1 receptors, although not constitutively present, are induced by endothelial cell stimulants such as the cytokines interleukin 1 and tumor necrosis factor α. An animal model[28] and theoretic considerations[29] indicate that the des-arg^9-bradykinin–B1 receptor interaction could contribute to the persistence of attacks of angioedema in

HAE, but we cannot yet test the hypothesis because a B1 receptor antagonist that could be used clinically is not available. Des-arg[9]-bradykinin, like bradykinin itself, is degraded to inactive peptide fragments by angiotensin-converting enzyme.[30]

THE PATHWAY(S) OF BRADYKININ FORMATION IN TYPES I AND II HEREDITARY ANGIOEDEMA

Bradykinin formation is typically initiated by negatively charged surfaces or macromolecules such as kaolin, glass (silicates), uric acid or pyrophosphate crystals, mast cell heparin, or platelet polyphosphate.[31] Dextran sulfate is an example of a soluble, negatively charged polymer that leads to factor XII activation as long as the polymer size can accommodate at least 2 factor XII molecules in proximity.[32] An autoactivation process occurs in which trace quantities of factor XIIa activates surface-bound factor XII to produce more factor XIIa, which is a slow process but one that accelerates with time. The second step is conversion of prekallikrein[33] to kallikrein by factor XIIa[34] followed by very rapid activation of remaining unactivated factor XII by kallikrein.[35,36] Kallikrein then digests high-molecular-weight kininogen to produce bradykinin[37] (**Fig. 3**). The digestion of factor XII by kallikrein produces 2 sequential forms of activated factor XII. The first, caused by digestion of an Arg-Val bond within a disulfide bridge produces factor XIIa (molecular weight of 80,000 Kd), which activates both prekallikrein to kallikrein and factor XI to factor XIa, each of which circulates as a complex with HK.[38,39] There is an important function of HK that relates to this binding because the rate of activation of both prekallikrein and factor XI are markedly increased,[40] which directly affects the rate of factor XII activation (ie, the rate of kallikrein formation to enzymatically activate factor XII).[41] The molar ratios are 1:1 (prekallikrein-HK) and 1:2 (factor XI-(HK)$_2$) because factor XI circulates as a dimer. Two subsequent cleavages in close proximity produces factor XIIf (fragment, molecular weight of 28,500–30,000) usually seen as a doublet on

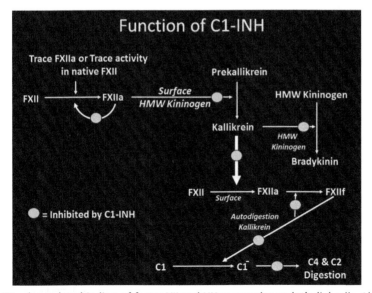

Fig. 3. Zinc-dependent binding of factor XII and HK to vascular endothelial cells. Although both bind to gC1qR, which is present in excess, there is preferential binding of factor XII to the complex of urokinase plasminogen activator receptor and cytokeratin 1, while HK binds primarily to the complex of gC1qR and cytokeratin 1. C1-INH, C1 inhibitor.

SDS gels, which readily converts prekallikrein to kallikrein,[33] but retains only minimal ability to activate factor XI because the surface binding site is lost. Factor XIIf is also the form of activated factor XII that activates the C1r subcomponent of complement[42] (see **Fig. 3**), which occurs during episodes of angioedema. At that time, C4 levels decrease further, often toward zero, and C2 levels diminish.[13] The plasma enzymes inhibited by C1-INH are the activated forms of C1r and C1s, both activated forms of factor XII (factor XIIa and factor XIIf; alternative nomenclature used is α factor XIIa and β factor XIIa, respectively), plasma kallikrein, coagulation factor XIa, and MASP I and MASP II of the lectin complement pathway. It is of interest that activated MASP I is elevated during attacks of HAE, which may relate to the severity of the clinical presentation[42] and MASP I can directly cleave HK to release bradykinin.[43] Its contribution to the actual pathogenesis of attacks is not yet clear. The fibrinolytic enzyme plasmin destroys C1-INH[36] and could contribute to pathogenesis by lowering C1-INH levels even further.

VASOPERMEABILITY OWING TO BRADYKININ

Bradykinin stimulates endothelial cell B2 receptors to cause vasodilatation and increase vascular permeability. Like histamine, the receptor density is most prominent along small venules. The effect is rapid but downregulated by internalization of the B2 receptor.[44] Vasodilators such as nitric oxide and prostacyclin and/or PGE_2 are secreted secondarily. The resultant effect is to stimulate adherens junctions between endothelial cells. The major protein of adherens junctions is VE cadherin (cadherins create zipperlike structures), which becomes phosphorylated at specific tyrosine residues and it is then internalized, ubiquinated, and eliminated. This leads to reversible opening of adherens cell junctions and plasma leakage.[45,46] In animal models, point mutations in these tyrosine residues inhibits bradykinin-induced vascular permeability. Phosphorylation of myosin light chain also can lead to retraction of actomyosin to open intercellular gaps.

The second bradykinin receptor, B-1, is not normally present, but is induced by inflammatory stimuli such as interleukin 1. Its ligand is a cleavage product of bradykinin, namely, des arg[9] bradykinin (C-terminal arginine has been removed), which can then function similarly to bradykinin. The B-1 receptor is not internalized readily; thus, its effects can be longer lasting and it possesses ligand-independent constitutive activity.[47] It has been suggested that its stimulation might relate to the location or duration of attacks of swelling.[28,29] Unfortunately, we do not have B-1 receptor antagonists that would allow one to test that possibility. Icatibant is a selective B-2 receptor antagonist with efficacy for acute episodes.

ASSEMBLY AND ACTIVATION OF THE BRADYKININ-FORMING CASCADE ON ENDOTHELIAL CELLS

The components of the plasma bradykinin-forming cascade bind to vascular endothelial cells[48] and in a zinc-dependent reaction. Binding involves the globular receptor for C1q (gC1qR),[49] which is present in excess, as well as bimolecular complexes of cytokeratin 1 with either gC1qR or with the urokinase plasminogen activator receptor.[50] **Fig. 4** depicts the binding of factor XII and HK to each cell surface molecular complex.

This model system led to new considerations regarding contact activation. Particularly noteworthy is that attachment of factor XII alone to the surface does not lead to significant activation,[51] but if the HK–prekallikrein complex binds, it activates without factor XII being present. This led to a series of observations, some in the fluid phase, and some requiring surface binding, as summarized in **Fig. 5** and **Box 1**. First, incubation of prekallikrein with HK in equimolar amounts in a nonphosphate buffer (eg, HEPES buffer) leads to stoichiometric cleavage of HK.[52] Prekallikrein has no active

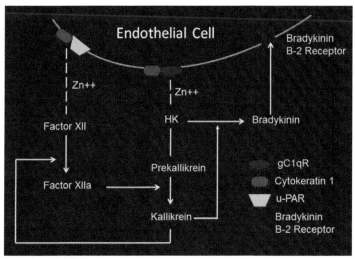

Fig. 4. Formation of bradykinin in hereditary angioedema, including the enzymatic steps inhibited by C1 inhibitor.

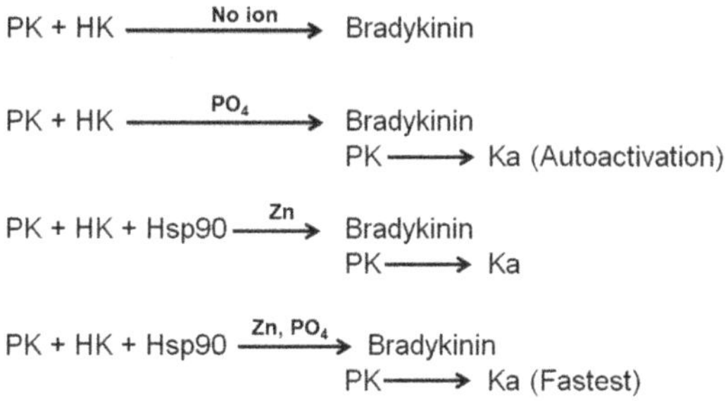

$$PK + HK \xrightarrow{\text{No ion}} Bradykinin$$

$$PK + HK \xrightarrow{PO_4} Bradykinin$$
$$PK \longrightarrow Ka \text{ (Autoactivation)}$$

$$PK + HK + Hsp90 \xrightarrow{Zn} Bradykinin$$
$$PK \longrightarrow Ka$$

$$PK + HK + Hsp90 \xrightarrow{Zn, PO_4} Bradykinin$$
$$PK \longrightarrow Ka \text{ (Fastest)}$$

Fig. 5. In vitro reactions observed with the prekallikrein-HK complex. HSP90, heat shock protein 90 Ka, kallikrein.

Box 1
Characteristics of PK-HK activity

1. PK is not an enzyme; the complex, however, is.

2. PK stoichiometrically cleaves HK in nonphosphate buffer and remains as PK. But plasma is phosphate based.

3. PK-HK autoactivates in phosphate buffer so PK becomes kallikrein and HK is cleaved.

4. Hsp90 + #2 → kallikrein.

5. Hsp90 accelerates #3.

site! Thus, we propose an induced site in prekallikrein upon binding to HK followed by HK cleavage to produce bradykinin. The evidence against even a trace of kallikrein being present is: (1) The reaction is indeed stoichiometric; for example, 5 molecules of prekallikrein bound to 50 molecules of HK cleaves only 5 HK. Kallikrein would cleave all of it. (2) The reaction is inhibited by corn trypsin inhibitor, which has no effect on kallikrein. (3) A peptide that prevents complex formation between prekallikrein and HK prevents any HK cleavage and the peptide has no effect on kallikrein. The situation changes in phosphate buffer (plasma buffer is phosphate). Then the prekallikrein–HK complex autoactivates and the product is kallikrein (ka) and cleaved HK as if activated factor XII were present. These stoichiometric reactions are inhibited completely in plasma by the presence of C1-INH.[52] But what happens if C1-INH is not present, as in HAE types I and II? We know that with incubation at 37°C, kallikrein forms and bradykinin evolves without any obvious initiating surface. We then took factor XII–deficient plasma, which does not activate when initiating surfaces are added, removed C1-INH by immunoadsorption, and found that the plasma activated and generated kallikrein activity, as did HAE plasma when incubated at 37°C.[53] Thus, the instability of HAE plasma that led to the in vitro identification of bradykinin as the likely mediator of HAE attacks (and disproved the existence of C-2 kinin)[18] is due to autoactivation of HK–prekallikrein and does not require factor XII.

However, these fluid-phase observations were actually preceded by studies of the activation of HK–prekallikrein bound to endothelial cells. The cell surface reactions were carried out in nonphosphate buffers so that prekallikrein is stable even if HK becomes cleaved. With time, endothelial cells secrete a substance(s) that converts prekallikrein to kallikrein within the complex. Two groups identified 2 differing molecules capable of doing this. One is heat shock protein-90 (HSP-90), a "stress" protein that has phosphatase activity but no proteolytic site (see **Fig. 5** and **Box 1**).[54] The other is prolylcarboxypeptidase, which produces angiotensin 1-7 from angiotensin II.[55] Its mechanism resembles that of HSP-90 in that it acts stoichiometrically, does not activate prekallikrein unless it is bound to HK, and is inhibited by corn trypsin inhibitor. Prolylcarboxypeptidase is an exopeptidase apparently functioning, in this instance, as an endopeptidase, and its active site is said to be necessary for conversion of prekallikrein–HK to kallikrein. HSP-90 has no proteolytic active site, which raises questions about a requirement for any active site other than that within prekallikrein–HK. Regardless, the HSP-90 mechanism seems clear. It forms a trimolecular complex with HK–prekallikrein that requires zinc ion and binds primarily to the HK.[56] In nonphosphate buffer, the prekallikrein is converted stiochiometrically to kallikrein; that is, the amount of kallikrein formed is directly proportional to the ratio of HSP-90 to the complex of HK–prekallikrein. The activation of the HK–prekallikrein complex by HSP-90 is inhibited by C1-INH or corn trypsin inhibitor. In a phosphate milieu, in which HK–prekallikrein generates kallikrein anyway, the addition of HSP-90 increase the activation rate. Most recently, we have demonstrated that the addition of HSP-90 directly to normal plasma activates prekallikrein to kallikrein and generates bradykinin,[53] so as to override the inhibitory effect of C1-INH on prekallikrein-HK.

Issues raised by these observations are as follows.

(1) Could attacks of HAE begin at the endothelial cell surface with activation of HK–prekallikrein first and then activate factor XII by the kallikrein thus produced?
(2) If HK–prekallikrein has an active site controlled by the presence of C1-INH, when an initiating factor XII binding surface is added, does activation start by factor XII autoactivation followed by the kallikrein feedback, as is generally believed, or could the site in HK–prekallikrein cleave and activate surface-bound factor XII first?

Regarding the first possibility, we have demonstrated that interleukin 1, tumor necrosis factor α, and estrogen all stimulate HSP-90 secretion by endothelial cells,[55] reminiscent of hormone and infectious influences on attacks of angioedema in HAE types I and II.

HEREDITARY ANGIOEDEMA WITH NORMAL C1 INHIBITOR: NEW FORMS OF HEREDITARY ANGIOEDEMA

This entity was described by Bork and colleagues[2] and Binkley and Davis[3] as a hereditary form of HAE with normal functional C1-INH that is strikingly prominent in women and strongly dependent on estrogen. A subpopulation of patients (perhaps one-third, depending on the country or region) has a mutation at threonine 309 with replacement by lysine (most commonly) or arginine. There are also rare cases of deletions, insertions, and duplications.[57,58] The lysine substitution eliminates an O-carbohydrate attachment site so that the mutant protein is somewhat less in molecular weight and visible on SDS gels as a doublet.[59] Because it is a "dominant" gene defect, most are heterozygotes with a 50/50 mix of normal and mutant proteins. Rare homozygous mutations have been reported.[60] At first, it was reported that incubation of plasma with low concentrations of dextran sulfate (in contrast with the typical amount used, eg, 10 μg/mL) leads to augmented activation of the entire cascade. This was attributed to the absent carbohydrate[59] and enhanced autoactivation of factor XII was assumed. Next, it was found that replacement of threonine with lys or arg yields a new plasmin cleavage site and the addition of plasmin leads to an increased rate of mutant factor XII activation relative to normal factor XII.[61] A coordinated event follows because cleavage at this site does not activate factor XII, but the product, a lower molecular weight factor XII (about 35 Kd) is cleaved and activated at the usual Arg-Val

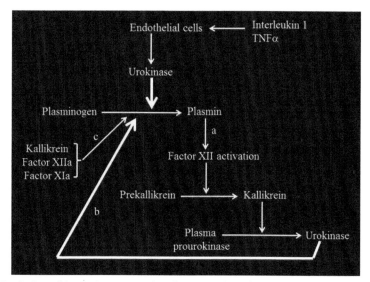

Fig. 6. Extrinsic and intrinsic sources of urokinase and/or plasmin, which may be critical for enzymatic activation of mutant factor XII in a subpopulation of patients with hereditary angioedema (HAE) and normal C1 inhibitor (type 3). [a] Important for activation of mutant factor XII (HAE with normal C1 inhibitor). [b] Major pathway for "intrinsic" activation of fibrinolysis. [c] Minor pathway for "intrinsic" activation of fibrinolysis; each enzyme is a weak plasminogen activator. TNFα, tumor necrosis factor α,

bond by either kallikrein or plasmin (Coen Maas, personal communication 2016). Both cleavages occur considerably faster than the rate of activation of normal factor XII; hence, enhanced activity is seen. Activation of factor XII by plasmin is not new; it was reported in 1971 by Kaplan and Austen[34] at a time when the activated forms of factor XII were first discovered. The product of the plasmin activation of mutant factor XII most closely resembles factor XIIf,[33] which lacks the surface binding site and activates prekallikrein readily with minimal activity on factor XI.

The source of plasmin could be exogenous for example, by secretion of urokinase or tissue plasminogen activator within tissues and diffusion into plasma, or generated through the intrinsic fibrinolytic cascade within plasma. The latter is relatively weak and it is unclear whether sufficient plasmin is generated in that fashion, particularly when all antifibrinolytic inhibitors are present. To that end, we have observed that interleukin 1 and tumor necrosis factor α , in the endothelial cell experiments as described, cause secretion of urokinase along with HSP-90, but not tissue plasminogen activator.[56] A proposed scheme by which enzymes of the fibrinolytic pathway can lead to bradykinin formation, particularly in HAE with factor XII mutation, is shown in **Fig. 6**. Further, subpopulations of HAE and normal C1-INH, with or without the factor XII mutation, have strikingly low levels of plasminogen activator inhibitor-2,[62] one of the plasma inhibitors of urokinase. Further work is in progress to define this subpopulation, but those with very low PAI-2 may have enhanced fibrinolysis and factor XII activation if urokinase is the initiating agonist.

REFERENCES

1. Donaldson V, Evans R. A biochemical abnormality in hereditary angioneurotic edema. Am J Med 1963;35:37–44.
2. Bork K, Barnstedt S, Koch P, et al. Hereditary angioedema with normal C1-inhibitor activity in women. Lancet 2000;356:213–7.
3. Binkley K, Davis A. Clinical, biochemical, and genetic characterization of a novel estrogen-dependent inherited form of angioedema. J Allergy Clin Immunol 2000; 106:546–50.
4. Dewald G, Bork K. Missense mutations in the coagulation factor XII (Hageman factor) gene in hereditary angioedema with normal C1 inhibitor. Biochem Biophys Res Commun 2006;343:1286–9.
5. Bork K, Wulff K, Hardt J, et al. Hereditary angioedema caused by missense mutations in the factor XII gene: clinical features, trigger factors, and therapy. J Allergy Clin Immunol 2009;124:129–34.
6. Pensky J, Levy L, Lepow I. Partial purification of a serum inhibitor of C'1-esterase. J Biol Chem 1961;236:1674–9.
7. Strang C, Siegel R, Phillips M, et al. Ultrastructure of the first component of human complement: electron microscopy of the crosslinked complex. Proc Natl Acad Sci U S A 1982;79:586–90.
8. Arlaud G, Villiers C, Chesne S, et al. Purified C1r: Some characteristics of its activation and subsequent proteolytic cleavage. Biochim Biophys Acta 1980;616: 116–29.
9. Ziccardi RJ. Spontaneous activation of the first component of human complement (C1) by an intramolecular autocatalytic mechanism. J Immunol 1982;128:2500–4.
10. Zuraw B. Clinical practice. Hereditary angioedema. N Engl J Med 2008;359: 1027–36.
11. Kramer J, Rosen F, Colten H, et al. Transinhibition of C1 inhibitor synthesis in type I hereditary angioneurotic edema. J Clin Immunol 1993;91:1258–62.

12. Patston P, Gettins P, Beechem J, et al. Mechanism of serpin action: evidence that C1 inhibitor functions as a suicide substrate. Biochemistry 1991;30:8876–82.

13. Austen K, Sheffer A. Detection of hereditary angioneurotic edema by demonstration of a reduction in the second component of human complement. N Engl J Med 1965;272:649–56.

14. Donaldson VH, Rosen FS, Bing DH. Role of the second component of complement (C2) and plasmin in kinin release in hereditary angioneurotic edema (H.A.N.E.) plasma. Trans Assoc Am Physicians 1977;90:174–83.

15. Klemperer MR, Donaldson VH, Rosen FS. Effect of C'1 esterase on vascular permeability in man: studies in normal and complement-deficient individuals and in patients with hereditary angioneurotic edema. J Clin Invest 1968;47:604–11.

16. Curd J, Prograis LJ, Cochrane C. Detection of active kallikrein in induced blister fluids of hereditary angioedema patients. N Engl J Med 1980;152:742–7.

17. Gigli I, Mason JW, Colman RW, et al. Interaction of plasma kallikrein with the C1 inhibitor. J Immunol 1970;104:574–81.

18. Fields T, Ghebrehiwet B, Kaplan AP. Kinin formation in hereditary angioedema plasma: evidence against kinin derivation from C2 and in support of "spontaneous" formation of bradykinin. J Allergy Clin Immunol 1983;72:54–60.

19. Smith M, Kerr M. Cleavage of the second component of complement by plasma proteases: implications in hereditary C1-inhibitor deficiency. Immunol 1985;56:561–70.

20. Shoemaker L, Schurman S, Donaldson V, et al. Hereditary angioneurotic oedema: characterization of plasma kinin and vascular permeability-enhancing activities. Clin Exp Immunol 1994;95:22–8.

21. Zahedi R, Bissler J, Davis A, et al. Unique C1 inhibitor dysfunction in a kindred without angioedema. II. Identification of an Ala443–>Val substitution and functional analysis of the recombinant mutant protein. J Clin Invest 1995;95:1299–305.

22. Nussberger J, Cugno M, Cicardi M, et al. Local bradykinin generation in hereditary angioedema. J Allergy Clin Immunol 1999;104:1321–2.

23. Han E, MacFarlane R, Mulligan A, et al. Increased vascular permeability in C1 inhibitor-deficient mice mediated by the bradykinin type 2 receptor. J Clin Invest 2002;8:1057–63.

24. Cicardi M, Banerji A, Bracho F. Icatibant, a new bradykinin receptor antagonist in hereditary angioedema. N Eng J Med 2010;363:532–41.

25. Cicardi M, Levy R, McNeil D. Ecallantide for the treatment of acute attacks in hereditary angioedema. N Eng J Med 2010;363:523–31.

26. Erdos E, Sloane G. An enzyme in human plasma that inactivates bradykinin and kallidins. Biochem Pharmacol 1962;11:585–92.

27. Skidgel R, Davis R, Tan F. Human carboxypeptidase M. Purification and characterization of a membrane-bound carboxypeptidase that cleaves peptide hormones. J Biol Chem 1989;264:2236–41.

28. Bossi F, Fischett F, Regoli D, et al. Novel pathogenic mechanism and therapeutic approaches to angioedema associated with C1 inhibitor deficiency. J Allergy Clin Immunol 2009;124:1303–10.

29. Hofman Z, Relan A, Zeerleder S, et al. Angioedema attacks in patients with hereditary angioedema: local manifestations of a systemic activation process. J Allergy Clin Immunol 2016;138:359–66.

30. Sheikh I, Kaplan A. Studies of the digestion of bradykinin, Lys-bradykinin, and des-Arg9-bradykinin by angiotensin converting enzyme. Biochem Pharmacol 1986;35:1951–6.

31. de Maat S, Maas C. Factor XII: form determines function. J Thromb Haemost 2016;14:1498–506.

32. Silverberg M, Diehl SV. The autoactivation of factor XII (Hageman factor) induced by low-Mr heparin and dextran sulphate. The effect of the Mr of the activating polyanion. Biochem J 1987;248:715–20.

33. Kaplan AP, Austen KF. A pre-albumin activator of prekallikrein. J Immunol 1970; 105:802–11.

34. Kaplan AP, Austen KF. A prealbumin activator of prekallikrein. II. Derivation of activators of prekallikrein from active Hageman factor by digestion with plasmin. J Exp Med 1971;133:696–712.

35. Revak S, Cochrane C, Bouma B, et al. Surface and fluid phase activities of two forms of activated Hageman factor produced during contact activation of plasma. J Exp Med 1978;147:719–29.

36. Wallace EM, Perkins SJ, Sim RB, et al. Degradation of C1-inhibitor by plasmin: implications for the control of inflammatory processes. Mol Med 1997;3:385–96.

37. Pierce J, Webster M. The purification and some properties of two different kallidinogen's from human plasma. In: Erdos E, Back N, Sicuteri F, editors. Hypotensive peptides. New York: Springer-Verlag; 1966. p. 130–8.

38. Mandle R, Colman R, Kaplan A. Identification of prekallikrein and high-molecular-weight kininogen as a complex in human plasma. Proc Natl Acad Sci U S A 1976; 73:4179–83.

39. Thompson R, Mandle RJ, Kaplan A. Association of factor XI and high molecular weight kininogen in human plasma. J Clin Invest 1977;60:1376–80.

40. Griffin JH, Cochrane CG. Mechanisms for the involvement of high molecular weight kininogen in surface-dependent reactions of Hageman factor. Proc Natl Acad Sci U S A 1976;73:2554–8.

41. Silverberg M, Nicoll J, Kaplan A. The mechanism by which the light chain of cleaved HMW-kininogen augments the activation of prekallikrein, factor XI and Hageman factor. Thromb Res 1980;20:173–89.

42. Hansen C, Csuka D, Munthe-Fog L, et al. The levels of the lectin pathway serine protease MASP-1 and its complex formation with C1 inhibitor are linked to the severity of hereditary angioedema. J Immunol 2015;195:3596–604.

43. Dobo J, Major B, Kekesi K, et al. Cleavage of kininogen and subsequent bradykinin release by the complement component: mannose-binding lectin-associated serine protease (MASP)-1. PLoS One 2011;6:e20036.

44. Enquist J, Skroder C, Whistler J, et al. Kinins promote B2 bradykinin receptor endocytosis and delay constitutive B1 receptor endocytosis. Mol Pharmacol 2007;71:494–507.

45. Orsenigo F, Giampietro C, Ferrari A, et al. Phosphorylation of VE-cadherin is modulated by haemodynamic forces and contributes to the regulation of vascular permeability in vivo. Nat Commun 2012;3:1208.

46. Bouillet L, Mannic T, Arboleas M, et al. Hereditary angioedema: key role for kallikrein and bradykinin in vascular endothelial-cadherin cleavage and edema formation. J Allergy Clin Immunol 2011;128:232–4.

47. Leeb-Lundberg L, Kang D, Lamb M, et al. The human B-1 bradykinin receptor exhibits high ligand-independent, constitutive activity. J Biol Chem 2001;276: 8785–92.

48. Schmaier AH, Kuo A, Lundberg D, et al. The expression of high molecular weight kininogen on human umbilical vein endothelial cells. J Biol Chem 1988;263: 16327–33.
49. Joseph K, Ghebrehiwet B, Peerschke EI, et al. Identification of the zinc-dependent endothelial cell binding protein for high molecular weight kininogen and factor XII: identity with the receptor that binds to the globular "heads" of C1q (gC1q-R). Proc Natl Acad Sci U S A 1996;93:8552–7.
50. Joseph K, Tholanikunnel B, Ghebrehiwet B, et al. Interaction of high molecular weight kininogen biding proteins on endothelial cells. Thromb Haemost 2004; 91:61–70.
51. Schmaier AH, Rojkjaer R, Shariat-Madar Z. Activation of the plasma kallikrein/kinin system on cells: a revised hypothesis. Thromb Haemost 1999;82:226–33.
52. Joseph K, Tholanikunnel B, Kaplan A. Factor XII-independent cleavage of high molecular weight kininogen by prekallikrein and inhibition by C1 inhibitor. J Allergy Clin Immunol 2009;124:143–9.
53. Joseph K, Kaplan A. Factor XII independent activation of the bradykinin-forming cascade: implications for the pathogenesis of hereditary angioedema types I and II. J Allergy Clin Immunol 2013;132:470–5.
54. Joseph K, Tholanikunnel B, Kaplan A. Heat shock protein 90 catalyzes activation of the prekallikrein-kininogen complex in the absence of factor XII. Proc Natl Acad Sci U S A 2002;99:896–900.
55. Shariat-Madar Z, Mahdi F, Schmaier A. Identification and characterization of pro-lylcarboxypeptidase as an endothelial cell prekallikrein activator. J Biol Chem 2002;277:17962–9.
56. Joseph K, Tholanikunnel B, Kaplan A. Cytokine and estrogen stimulation of endothelial cells augment activation of the prekallikrein-high molecular weight kininogen complex: Implications for hereditay angioedema (HAE). J Allergy Clin Immunol 2016. [Epub ahead of print].
57. Bork K, Wulff K, Meinke P. A novel mutation in the coagulation factor 12 gene in subjects with hereditary angioedema and normal C1 inhibitor. Clin Immunol 2011; 141:31–5.
58. Kiss N, Barabas E, Varnai K, et al. Novel duplication in the F12 gene in a patient with recurrent angioedema. Clin Immunol 2013;149:142–5.
59. Bjorkqvist J, de Maat S, Lewandrowski U, et al. Defective glycosylation of coagulation factor XII underlies hereditary angioedema type III. J Clin Invest 2015;125: 3132–46.
60. Grumach A, Stieber C, Veronez C, et al. Homozygosity for a factor XII mutation in one female and one male patient with hereditary angioedema. Allergy 2016;71: 119–23.
61. de Maat S, Bjorkqvist J, Suffritti C, et al. Plasmin is a natural trigger for bradykinin production in hereditary angioedema with factor XII mutation. J Allergy Clin Immunol 2016;138:1414–23.
62. Joseph K, Tholanikunnel B, Wolf B, et al. Deficiency of plasminogen activator inhibitor 2 in plasma of patients with hereditary angioedema with normal C1 inhibitor levels. J Allergy Clin Immunol 2015;137:1822–9.

Laboratory Approaches for Assessing Contact System Activation

Sandra C. Christiansen, MD[a], Bruce L. Zuraw, MD[a,b],*

KEYWORDS

- Contact system • Hereditary angioedema • C1 inhibitor • Bradykinin • C4
- C1 inhibitor complexes • Vascular permeability

KEY POINTS

- Activation of the plasma contact system generates bradykinin and causes swelling in hereditary angioedema (HAE) due to C1 inhibitor (C1INH) deficiency (HAE-C1INH), HAE associated with factor XII (FXII) mutations, and acquired C1INH deficiency (AC1D).
- Bradykinin is suspected to be the mediator of swelling in several other forms of angioedema, such as HAE of unknown type, idiopathic nonhistaminergic angioedema, and angioedema associated with inhibitors of kininases.
- Laboratory tests to detect activation of the contact system and generation of bradykinin remain limited to research settings at the current time.

INTRODUCTION

Angioedema is a common clinical finding that can reflect multiple underlying pathophysiologic mechanisms. It is the physical manifestation of fluid movement from the blood vessel into the interstitial fluid that occurs as a consequence of transiently increased vascular permeability. Unlike hydrostatic or oncotic causes of edema, angioedema results from the action of mediators on endothelial cells that disrupt the adherens junction, resulting in vascular leak.[1] Histamine, cysteinyl leukotrienes, and bradykinin are recognized as the principal biologic mediators of swelling.[2] A majority of angioedema cases are thought to involve mast cell activation, triggering the release of histamine and other mediators, such as leukotrienes.[3] Less frequently, angioedema is linked to the generation of bradykinin. Because the prognosis and treatment of bradykinin-mediated angioedema are markedly different from those of histamine-mediated or leukotriene-mediated angioedema, it is of considerable clinical

[a] Department of Medicine, University of California, 9500 Gilman Drive, Mailcode 0732, La Jolla, CA 92093, USA; [b] San Diego Veterans Administration Healthcare System, Medicine Service, 3350 La Jolla Village Drive, San Diego, CA 92161, USA
* Corresponding author. Department of Medicine, University of California, 9500 Gilman Drive, Mailcode 0732, La Jolla, CA 92093, USA.
E-mail address: bzuraw@ucsd.edu

Immunol Allergy Clin N Am 37 (2017) 527–539
http://dx.doi.org/10.1016/j.iac.2017.04.008
0889-8561/17/© 2017 Elsevier Inc. All rights reserved.

importance to identify whether angioedema is mast cell mediated (often called hista-minergic) or bradykinin mediated. This article reviews the forms of angioedema that are likely bradykinin mediated and discusses the laboratory approaches for establishing a diagnosis.

BRADYKININ-MEDIATED ANGIOEDEMA

The kallikrein-kinin system consists of proteases (kallikreins) that cleave their substrate (kininogens) to release bioactive kinin. There are 2 primary kallikreins, tissue kallikrein and plasma kallikrein (PK), which are immunologically and functionally distinct. Tissue kallikrein is widely distributed in mammalian tissues and releases Lys-bradykinin (BK) from low-molecular-weight kininogen. To date, there is no evidence that tissue kallikrein participates in angioedema. On the other hand, there is substantial evidence showing that PK is involved in bradykinin-mediated angioedema (See Allen P. Kaplan and Kusumam Joseph's article, "Pathogenesis of Hereditary Angioedema: the Role of the Bradykinin Forming Cascade," in this issue).

Activation of the contact system results in the generation of bradykinin, a biologic mediator of enhanced endothelial permeability. Bradykinin-mediated vascular leakage in susceptible individuals can trigger attacks of angioedema typified by nonpitting asymmetric tissue swelling. There is strong evidence that implicates activation of the contact system and generation of bradykinin in the pathogenesis of swelling in HAE-C1INH. The evidence for a role of contact system activation and bradykinin in HAE with normal C1INH (HAE-nl-C1INH) is highly suggestive but currently less clearly delineated. The evidence for both forms of HAE is summarized.

Role of Bradykinin in Hereditary Angioedema due to C1 Inhibitor Deficiency

Landerman and colleagues[4] reported in 1962 that plasma from patients with HAE failed to inhibit PK and plasma dilution factor—now known to be FXII. One year later, Donaldson and Evans[5] established that C1INH activity was absent in patients with HAE, thus providing the definitive biochemical explanation for the cause of type I HAE. Soon thereafter, Rosen and colleagues[6] described a group of HAE patients who had normal plasma C1INH protein levels but lacked C1INH functional activity, thereby defining type II HAE.

C1INH is the major inhibitor of both active PK and active FXII of the contact system cascade.[7] The genesis of swelling in HAE types I and II has been established to evolve from the generation of bradykinin, engagement with the constitutively expressed B2-receptor on endothelial cells, and resultant vascular leak. Acceptance of the central role of the contact system in HAE was founded on series of observations recently reviewed.[8] In 1980 Curd and colleagues[9] detected active PK in the interstitial fluid from patients with HAE followed in 1982 by sequencing bradykinin as the permeability inducing factor.[10] This observation was extended by Fields and colleagues,[11] demonstrating that bradykinin, not C2 kinin, was responsible for vascular permeability. Further proof of the central role of contact system activation in HAE included the consumption of high-molecular-weight kininogen (HMWK) and cleavage of PK during attacks[12] as well as evidence that HMWK was cleaved during HAE attacks.[13–15]

Subsequently, plasma BK levels in HAE-C1INH subjects were shown significantly increased during attacks and normal or slightly increased during remission.[16,17] Most recently, well-controlled clinical trials have shown that the PK inhibitor ecallantide as well as the bradykinin B2-receptor antagonist icatibant are effective in the treatment of HAE-C1INH.[18,19] The increased circulating BK levels during attacks have been claimed to originate from the site of angioedema.[17] Based on the catabolism of bradykinin in both animal and human models, this has been interpreted as a systemic activation process of the contact system with local manifestation of disease.[20]

Although many of the attacks in HAE are unpredictable, stress, infection, and trauma have all been implicated,[21] which can be linked to the candidate physiologic activators (discussed previously). Enzymatic activation of PK on endothelial cells has also been associated with heat shock protein 90,[22] which is secreted during cellular stress. Heat shock protein 90, which lacks enzymatic activity, can interact with plasma prekallikrein (PPK) in complex with HMWK in the presence of Zinc (Zn+) to convert PPK to PK.[23] The stoichiometric generation of PK from PPK could thus play an initiating role in contact system activation and attacks of angioedema.

Role of Bradykinin in Hereditary Angioedema with Normal C1 Inhibitor

In 2000, Bork and colleagues[24] and Binkley and colleagues[25] independently described a form of HAE characterized by normal C1INH antigenic and functional levels. Thus, HAE is now classified as either HAE-C1INH or HAE-nl-C1INH. A minority (approximately 25% in Europe but much less in the United States) of patients with HAE-nl-C1INH were subsequently shown to have mutations in exon 9 of the F12 gene.[26] Based on this, HAE-nl-C1INH has been subdivided into HAE-XII for patients with an F12 mutation and HAE-nl-C1INH unknown type (HAE-U) for patients without an F12 mutation.[27] The mutant FXII has been shown to confer an increased ease of activation of the contact cascade.[28] FXII HAE mutations seem to create new sites susceptible to enzymatic cleavage by plasmin, thereby escaping inhibition by C1INH and providing a pathway for bradykinin formation.[29] Polymorphisms associated with lower levels of both aminopeptidase P and angiotensin-converting enzyme (ACE), enzymes involved in bradykinin degradation, have been reported in subjects with the FXII mutation.[30] As is the case for HAE types I and II, there is substantial evidence for HAE-nl-C1INH that the swelling is mediated by kinin generation.[31,32] Successful treatment with a B2-antagonist has also provided putative evidence that bradykinin is the mediator of swelling.[33]

Role of Bradykinin in Other Forms of Angioedema

Bradykinin is also thought to be the primary mediator of swelling in several other types of angioedema. AC1D is clinically nearly indistinguishable from HAE-C1INH. The pathophysiologic consequences of C1INH deficiency would be expected to be similar whether the deficiency is hereditary or acquired. Not surprisingly, angioedema attacks in patients with AC1D has been shown accompanied by elevated plasma bradykinin levels.[16]

Another group of patients is defined by angioedema unresponsive to antihistamines who have normal C1INH, normal FXII, and no family history of angioedema. This group has been called, idiopathic angioedema unresponsive to antihistamines.[34] Many of these patients do respond to bradykinin-targeted therapy, and the angioedema in these patients may be bradykinin mediated. Because of the low penetrance seen in HAE-U, and the lack of a genetic marker, it is possible that these patients are actually part of the HAE-U group.

Angioedema has additionally been reported to occur in patients treated with a variety of drugs that act on the renin-angiotensin system, especially ACE inhibitors (ACEIs) (See Cosby Stone and Nancy J. Brown's article, "ACE-Inhibitor and Other Drug-Associated Angioedema," in this issue). Plasma levels of bradykinin were shown to be very high at the time of swelling in ACE angioedema (ACEI-AE) but returned to normal after withdrawal of the drug and resolution of the angioedema.[16] In 3 other patients with a history of ACEI-AE, bradykinin levels were high during ACEI treatment.[35]

Although anecdotal clinical experience has suggested that icatibant and ecallantide have beneficial effects in the treatment of ACEI-AE, randomized clinical studies have yielded mixed but not encouraging results—possibly due to the logistical challenges involved in treating this form of angioedema. One randomized double-blind clinical trial show that icatibant was effective in treating ACEI-AE if given early in the attack.[36] Two subsequent studies failed to show any benefit for icatibant.[37]

LABORATORY DIAGNOSIS OF ANGIOEDEMA

Early recognition and proper diagnosis of bradykinin-mediated angioedema are essential to avoid excess morbidity and potentially fatal outcomes from the disease. Clinically, a high index of suspicion should be maintained in cases of recurrent angioedema in absence of urticaria or unexplained spontaneously reversible abdominal pain. Ultimately, clinical suspicion must be confirmed by appropriate laboratory testing (**Table 1**).

Angioedema Associated with C1 Inhibitor Deficiency

Laboratory measurements are targeted for both activation of the contact system and importantly the complement cascade for which C1 inhibitor is a primary regulatory

Table 1
Clinical situations where laboratory testing for contact system activation may be most useful

Test	Major Advantages	Major Disadvantages
C1INH level	Easy to perform; critical for diagnosis of HAE-C1INH and AC1D	Antigenic level may give deceiving result; can be false positive or negative; can be influenced by treatment
C4 level	Important for diagnosis of HAE-C1INH and AC1D	Substantial variability in the general population; can be influenced by treatment
Protease-inhibitor complexes	Easy to measure as biomarker of contact system activation; may be useful as novel assay for C1INH function	Complexes are short-lived in vivo; subject to ex vivo artifact; may be artificially low in C1INH deficiency
Cleaved protease	Directly reflects contact system activation	Difficult to measure, requires immunoblotting or antibody to neoepitope; subject to ex vivo artifact
Kallikrein activity	Simple and straightforward assay; able to be standardized	Spontaneous activity subject to ex vivo artifact; activity not completely specific
Cleaved HMWK	Stable biomarker of contact system activation; moderately sensitive	Difficult to measure, requires immunoblotting or antibody to neoepitope; subject to ex vivo artifact
Bradykinin level	Theoretically the best biomarker of contact system activation	Very difficult to measure; extremely short half-life of peptide; subject to ex vivo artifact
Fibrinolysis	Easy to measure; may reflect primary or secondary events in contact system activation	Very nonspecific and subject to variability

protein.[7] For HAE-C1INH, commercially available laboratory evaluation is straightforward with type I HAE characterized by low C4 and C1INH antigenic levels whereas type II HAE is characterized by low C4 levels and low C1INH functional levels.[21] There can be some variability in the measurement of C4 levels, which in particular can confound the diagnosis between attacks or during treatment with attenuated androgen therapy resulting in normalization of the C4.[38] Although not commercially available, the most sensitive test is a C4d/C4 ratio reflecting complement system activation in the setting of deficient C1INH functional levels. A normal C4d/C4 ratio excludes CIINH deficiency, even if the patient is not actively swelling or is receiving attenuated androgen treatment.[39] AC1D typically presents with low C4 and C1INH levels but can be distinguished from HAE-C1INH by the later age of onset, lack of a family history of angioedema, and often a low C1q level.[40]

Bradykinin-Mediated Angioedema with Normal C1 Inhibitor

The diagnosis of HAE-nl-C1INH presently rests on a collection of criteria, including clinical expression of disease, hereditary pattern, and response to therapy.[27] Unlike for HAE-C1INH, there is no available laboratory confirmation or clear-cut biomarker. HAE-nl-C1INH is characterized not only by normal C4 and C1INH levels but also by a lack of SERPING1 mutations. A minority of HAE-nl-C1INH patients have a mutation in exon 9 of the F12 gene.[26] A diagnosis of ACEI-associated angioedema or ARB-associated angioedema is typically a diagnosis of exclusion, which is confirmed if the angioedema remits after stopping the drug.

BIOMARKERS OF CONTACT SYSTEM ACTIVATION

Biomarkers can be defined as objective measures that reflect a biologic process. Validated biomarkers of contact system activation would infer whether or not bradykinin had been generated and could thus be extremely helpful in characterizing angioedema as either bradykinin mediated or not. Beyond their use for accurate diagnosis, biomarkers of contact system activation may be valuable in patients with a known diagnosis of bradykinin-mediated angioedema to understand whether specific symptoms are related to an angioedema attack. A variety of different potential biomarkers of contact system activation are summarized, describing the assay, its interpretation, and its limitations.

Measurement of C1 Inhibitor Levels

C1INH is the major inhibitor of the early complement proteases C1r, C1s, and the mannose-binding lectin-associated serine protease (MASP) 1 and 2 as well as the contact-system proteases, PK and activated FXII.[7] C1INH is also a minor inhibitor of plasmin and factor XIa. In the absence of sufficient C1INH levels, activation of target proteases is enhanced. Because of its key role in inhibiting the contact system proteases, low C1INH levels are a reasonable surrogate marker for contact system activation. Although it is accepted that the fundamental cause of HAE-C1INH is a deficiency of functional C1INH, it has proved difficult to show that C1INH levels directly correlate with disease severity although 1 article reported that C1INH functional levels correlated with overall HAE severity.[41]

C1INH levels can be measured by assessing total antigenic protein levels or by assessing C1INH functional levels. In type I HAE and AC1D, C1INH antigenic levels are reduced, and this has been a key component in the diagnosing these forms of angioedema. C1INH antigenic levels are normal in type II HAE and, therefore, this diagnosis depends on the measurement of C1INH function.

At least 3 different ways to assess C1INH function have been described. The ability of C1INH to inhibit active C1s in a solid-phase ELISA assay is the most commonly used laboratory test for C1INH function. This test, however, can show false normal values,[42] and caution should be used in interpreting a low normal result. The chromogenic C1INH functional assay measures the ability of C1INH to inhibit C1s activity in a solution phase assay. This test is more sensitive than the ELISA assay but can show falsely low C1INH functional levels if the plasma was not prepared and handled carefully. The third assay is the measurement of C1INH function determined by its binding to immobilized activated FXII or kallikrein.[43] This assay has the advantage of directly measuring the ability of C1INH to complex with the relevant contact system proteases; however, this test is not yet commercially available.

C4 Levels

Measurement of C4 levels is a routine component of the standard diagnostic panel for HAE-C1INH and AC1D. Although not 100% sensitive when measured at a time a patient is not swelling, the C4 level is invariably decreased during attacks of angioedema in patients with HAE-C1INH. When FXIIa is generated, it can be further cleaved by kallikrein to generate B-FXIIa (also known as FXIIf), which can efficiently activate C4.[44] Because of this, measurement of C4 during an attack of angioedema might have some usefulness even in the situation where C1INH is normal.

Measurement of Protease-Inhibitor Complexes

A more direct biomarker for contact system activation is the measurement of in vivo formed protease-inhibitor complexes. C1INH is a member of the serpin superfamily of inhibitors.[45] Like other serine protease inhibitors, it has been described as a molecular mousetrap, with a reactive mobile loop critical for their functional activity.[46] The reactive center is fully exposed in the aqueous environment. Target proteases attack and cleave the Arg^{444}-Thr^{445} bond within the C1INH reactive mobile loop leading to a thermodynamically favorable conformational rearrangement that irreversibly traps the protease within the C1INH molecule.[47] C1INH thus functions as a suicide inactivator of PK of the contact system, and detection of these complexes could serve as a biomarker of contact system activation.

C1INH forms SDS-stable complexes with FXIIa and kallikrein.[48,49] Sandwich-type ELISA assays developed to detect these complexes were able to sensitively measure ex vivo activation of the contact system.[50,51] Attempts to use these assays to measure in vivo activation of the contact system, however, showed modest increases in protease-inhibitor complexes despite substantial in vivo activation,[52,53] including during HAE attacks (Zuraw, unpublished data). Presumably, these complexes are cleared rapidly in vivo, preventing a significant increase to be measured.[54–56] A a specific serpin-enzyme complex receptor was identified on human hepatoma cells and monocytes.[57] When samples are drawn rapidly (5–15 minutes) after a discrete activation of the contact system, increased kallikrein-C1INH and FXIIa-C1INH levels can be measured.[58] C1INH also forms complexes with both MASP-1 and MASP-2.[59,60] The relevance of this stems from MASPs reported as capable of generating bradykinin from HMWK.[61] An additional problem with measuring protease-C1INH levels in HAE-C1INH is that the low levels of functional C1INH limit the sensitivity of these assays[62]; however, this would not be a problem in bradykinin-mediated angioedema not associated with C1INH deficiency.

Cleavage of Zymogen Proteases

Activation of the contact system is associated with cleavage of the zymogen proteases prekallikrein and FXII into their active proteolytic forms, kallikrein and FXII. This cleavage can be monitored by immunoblotting based on changes in the migration of the specific bands. A monoclonal antibody that recognizes only FXIIa or bFXIIa has been reported[63] and could be used to detect activated FXII without immunoblotting.[64] It is likely, however, that these proteases do not circulate for long before they are complexed to inhibitors or cleared.

High-Molecular-Weight Kininogen Cleavage

Coagulant levels of HMWK were shown to fall during severe attacks of angioedema in patients with HAE-C1INH.[12] Detection of HMWK cleavage by immunoblotting was first reported in 1986 and was found a highly sensitive marker for HAE-C1INH attacks.[13–15] During HAE-C1INH attacks, HMWK was almost completely cleaved.[65] Measurement of HMWK cleavage in remission samples has also been shown to correlate with HAE-C1INH disease severity.[66] HMWK cleavage was also reported to be increased in women with HAE-nl-C1INH.[67] Although promising for use as a biomarker of contact system activation, measurement of HMWK cleavage remains laborious and subject to significant potential artifact from ex vivo contact system activation during blood drawing, processing, and storage. Although attacks of HAE are localized to 1 or more sites of swelling the degree of HMWK cleavage measured seems to point toward a systemic activation process.[20]

Bradykinin Levels

Direct measurement of bradykinin could be an ideal test to confirm the involvement of bradykinin in angioedema; however, the short half-life of bradykinin in plasma plus the technical difficulties in measuring bradykinin have limited the applicability of this technique. Using scrupulous attention to the process of preparing the samples, elevated levels of bradykinin were detected during attacks of angioedema in patients with HAE-C1INH, AC1D, and ACEI-associated angioedema.[16,17,68] Measurement of bradykinin metabolites that have a longer circulating half-life than bradykinin may be more feasible, although at present these assays are highly specialized.[69,70]

Measurement of Kallikrein Activity

Kallikrein amidolytic activity can be readily measured using synthetic substrates. Several reports have described increased kallikrein activity in the plasma of patients with HAE-C1INH[66] and HAE-nl-C1INH.[32] Although promising, these assays need to be validated and confirmed.

Other Assays

Although it has yet to be confirmed as a reliable biomarker, Joseph and colleagues[71] showed that HAE-XII and HAE-U patients have markedly reduced plasminogen activator inhibitor type 2 levels compared with normal controls or patients with HAE-C1INH. Activation of the FXII-kallikrein pathway results in secondary activation of the fibrinolytic system. Elevations of D-dimers and plasmin-α_2-antiplasmain complexes have been consistently observed in HAE-C1INH.[65,72,73]

SUMMARY

The role of contact system activation and generation of bradykinin have been clearly established for HAE-C1INH (**Figs. 1** and **2**). Insights continue to emerge regarding the

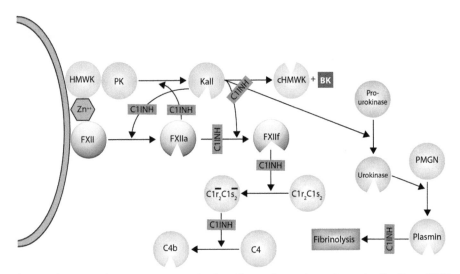

Fig. 1. Schematic of contact system activation. Figure shows the reciprocal activation of PPK (PK) and FXII to kallikrein (Kall) and FXIIa with cleavage of HMWK to cleaved HMWK (cHMWK) and release of bradykinin (BK). Kallikrein also activates prourokinase to urokinase, which activates plasminogen (PMGN) to plasmin. B-FXIIa (FXIIf) can activate the classical complement pathway. Steps inhibited by C1INH as shown.

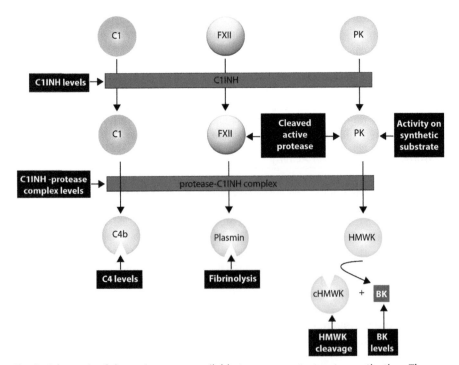

Fig. 2. Schematic of the major assays available to assess contact system activation. The contact system is shown in an abstracted manner that shows the different levels of activation and cleavage. The events measured by each of the laboratory assays are shown by black boxes with white text and arrows.

factors governing local expression of what is fundamentally a systemic disease. In experimental studies, C1INH-protease complexes, levels of functional C1INH, PK activation, and cleavage of HMWK have all been linked with disease activity. For HAE-nl-C1INH, there is compelling evidence as well for contact system activation and bradykinin generation underlying enhanced vascular permeability and angioedema attacks. Recent work has provided key insights as to the role of FXII genetic mutations and plasmin as an activator of the contact system, which eludes C1INH. To build on these findings and establish a reliable biomarker for HAE-nl-C1INH and other forms of bradykinin-mediated angioedema with normal C1INH will be the focus of ongoing research in years to come. The ability to confirm contact system activation would have important implications for the diagnosis and effective management of angioedema.

REFERENCES

1. Dejana E, Giampietro C. Vascular endothelial-cadherin and vascular stability. Curr Opin Hematol 2012;19:218–23.
2. Zuraw BL, Bernstein JA, Lang DM, et al. A focused parameter update: hereditary angioedema, acquired C1 inhibitor deficiency, and angiotensin-converting enzyme inhibitor-associated angioedema. J Allergy Clin Immunol 2013;131: 1491–3.
3. Altman K, Chang C. Pathogenic intracellular and autoimmune mechanisms in urticaria and angioedema. Clin Rev Allergy Immunol 2013;45:47–62.
4. Landerman NS, Webster ME, Becker EL, et al. Hereditary angioneurotic edema. II. Deficiency of inhibitor for serum globulin permeability factor and/or plasma kallikrein. J Allergy 1962;33:330–41.
5. Donaldson VH, Evans RR. A biochemical abnormality in hereditary angioneurotic edema: absence of serum inhibitor of C'1- esterase. Am J Med 1963;35:37–44.
6. Rosen FS, Charache P, Pensky J, et al. Hereditary angioneurotic edema: two genetic variants. Science 1965;148:957–8.
7. Davis AE 3rd. Mechanism of angioedema in first complement component inhibitor deficiency. Immunol Allergy Clin North Am 2006;26:633–51.
8. Zuraw BL, Christiansen SC. HAE pathophysiology and underlying mechanisms. Clin Rev Allergy Immunol 2016;51:216–29.
9. Curd JG, Prograis L Jr, Cochrane CG. Detection of active kallikein in induced blister fluids of hereditary angioedema patients. J Exp Med 1980;152:742–7.
10. Curd JG, Yelvington M, Burridge N, et al. Generation of bradykinin during incubation of hereditary angioedema plasma. Mol Immunol 1982;19:1365.
11. Fields T, Ghebrehiwet B, Kaplan AP. Kinin formation in hereditary angioedema plasma: evidence against kinin derivation from C2 and in support of "spontaneous" formation of bradykinin. J Allergy Clin Immunol 1983;72:54–60.
12. Schapira M, Silver LD, Scott CF, et al. Prekallikrein activation and high- molecular-weight kininogen consumption in hereditary angioedema. N Engl J Med 1983; 308:1050–4.
13. Berrettini M, Lammle B, White T, et al. Detection of in vitro and in vivo cleavage of high molecular weight kininogen in human plasma by immunoblotting with monoclonal antibodies. Blood 1986;68:455–62.
14. Zuraw BL, Lammle B, Sugimoto S, et al. Cleavage of high molecular weight kininogen in plasma during attacks of angioedema in hereditary angioedema. J Allergy Clin Immunol 1987;79:177.

15. Lammle B, Zuraw BL, Heeb MJ, et al. Detection and quantitation of cleaved and uncleaved high molecular weight kininogen in plasma by ligand blotting with radiolabeled plasma prekallikrein or factor XI. Thromb Haemost 1988;59:151–61.

16. Nussberger J, Cugno M, Amstutz C, et al. Plasma bradykinin in angio-oedema. Lancet 1998;351:1693–7.

17. Nussberger J, Cugno M, Cicardi M, et al. Local bradykinin generation in hereditary angioedema. J Allergy Clin Immunol 1999;104:1321–2.

18. Cicardi M, Banerji A, Bracho F, et al. Icatibant, a new bradykinin-receptor antagonist, in hereditary angioedema. N Engl J Med 2010;363:532–41.

19. Cicardi M, Levy RJ, McNeil DL, et al. Ecallantide for the treatment of acute attacks in hereditary angioedema. N Engl J Med 2010;363:523–31.

20. Hofman ZLM, Relan A, Zeerleeder S, et al. Angioedema attacks of hereditary angioedema: local manifestations of a systemic activation process. J Allergy Clin Immunol 2016;138(2):359–66, in revision.

21. Zuraw BL. Clinical practice. Hereditary angioedema. N Engl J Med 2008;359: 1027–36.

22. Joseph K, Tholanikunnel BG, Kaplan AP. Heat shock protein 90 catalyzes activation of the prekallikrein-kininogen complex in the absence of factor XII. Proc Natl Acad Sci U S A 2002;99:896–900.

23. Joseph K, Tholanikunnel BG, Bygum A, et al. Factor XII-independent activation of the bradykinin-forming cascade: implications for the pathogenesis of hereditary angioedema types I and II. J Allergy Clin Immunol 2013;132(2):470–5.

24. Bork K, Barnstedt SE, Koch P, et al. Hereditary angioedema with normal C1-inhibitor activity in women. Lancet 2000;356:213–7.

25. Binkley KE, Davis A 3rd. Clinical, biochemical, and genetic characterization of a novel estrogen- dependent inherited form of angioedema. J Allergy Clin Immunol 2000;106:546–50.

26. Dewald G, Bork K. Missense mutations in the coagulation factor XII (Hageman factor) gene in hereditary angioedema with normal C1 inhibitor. Biochem Biophys Res Commun 2006;343:1286–9.

27. Zuraw BL, Bork K, Binkley KE, et al. Hereditary angioedema with normal C1 inhibitor function: consensus of an international expert panel. Allergy Asthma Proc 2012;33(Suppl 1):S145–56.

28. Bjorkqvist J, de Maat S, Lewandrowski U, et al. Defective glycosylation of coagulation factor XII underlies hereditary angioedema type III. J Clin Invest 2015;125: 3132–46.

29. de Maat S, Bjorkqvist J, Suffritti C, et al. Plasmin is a natural trigger for bradykinin production in patients with hereditary angioedema with factor XII mutations. J Allergy Clin Immunol 2016;138(5):1414–23.e9.

30. Duan QL, Binkley K, Rouleau GA. Genetic analysis of factor XII and bradykinin catabolic enzymes in a family with estrogen-dependent inherited angioedema. J Allergy Clin Immunol 2009;123:906–10.

31. Hentges F, Hilger C, Kohnen M, et al. Angioedema and estrogen-dependent angioedema with activation of the contact system. J Allergy Clin Immunol 2009;123: 262–4.

32. Defendi F, Charignon D, Ghannam A, et al. Enzymatic assays for the diagnosis of bradykinin-dependent angioedema. PLoS One 2013;8:e70140.

33. Vitrat-Hincky V, Gompel A, Dumestre-Perard C, et al. Type III hereditary angio-oedema: clinical and biological features in a French cohort. Allergy 2010;65: 1331–6.

34. Bork K, Wulff K, Witzke G, et al. Antihistamine-resistant angioedema in women with negative family history: estrogens and F12 gene mutations. Am J Med 2013;126:1142 e9-14.

35. Nussberger J, Cugno M, Cicardi M. Bradykinin-mediated angioedema. N Engl J Med 2002;347:621–2.

36. Bas M, Greve J, Stelter K, et al. A randomized trial of icatibant in ACE-inhibitor-induced angioedema. N Engl J Med 2015;372:418–25.

37. Straka BT, Ramirez CE, Byrd JB, et al. Effect of bradykinin receptor antagonism on ACE inhibitor-associated angioedema. J Allergy Clin Immunol 2016 [pii:S0091-6749(16)31376-8].

38. Gelfand JA, Sherins RJ, Alling DW, et al. Treatment of hereditary angioedema with danazol. N Engl J Med 1976;295:1444–8.

39. Zuraw BL, Sugimoto S, Curd JG. The value of rocket immunoelectrophoresis for C4 activation in the evaluation of patients with angioedema or C1-inhibitor deficiency. J Allergy Clin Immunol 1986;78:1115–20.

40. Cicardi M, Zingale LC, Pappalardo E, et al. Autoantibodies and lymphoproliferative diseases in acquired C1-inhibitor deficiencies. Medicine (Baltimore) 2003;82: 274–81.

41. Csuka D, Fust G, Farkas H, et al. Parameters of the classical complement pathway predict disease severity in hereditary angioedema. Clin Immunol 2011;139:85–93.

42. Wagenaar-Bos IG, Drouet C, Aygoren-Pursun E, et al. Functional C1-inhibitor diagnostics in hereditary angioedema: assay evaluation and recommendations. J Immunol Methods 2008;338:14–20.

43. Joseph K, Bains S, Tholanikunnel BG, et al. A novel assay to diagnose hereditary angioedema utilizing inhibition of bradykinin-forming enzymes. Allergy 2015;70: 115–9.

44. Ghebrehiwet B, Silverberg M, Kaplan AP. Activation of the classical pathway of complement by Hageman factor fragment. J Exp Med 1981;153:665–76.

45. Tosi M, Duponchel C, Bourgarel P, et al. Molecular cloning of human C1 inhibitor: sequence homologies with alpha 1-antitrypsin and other members of the serpins superfamily. Gene 1986;42:265–72.

46. Huber R, Carrell RW. Implications of the three-dimensional structure of alpha1-antitrypsin for structure and function of serpins. Biochemistry 1989;28: 8951–66.

47. Gettins PG. Serpin structure, mechanism, and function. Chem Rev 2002;102: 4751–804.

48. Zuraw BL, Curd JG. Demonstration of modified inactive first component of complement (C1) inhibitor in the plasmas of C1 inhibitor-deficient patients. J Clin Invest 1986;78:567–75.

49. de Agostini A, Lijnen HR, Pixley RA, et al. Inactivation of factor XII active fragment in normal plasma. Predominant role of C-1-inhibitor. J Clin Invest 1984;73:1542–9.

50. Kaplan AP, Gruber B, Harpel PC. Assessment of Hageman factor activation in human plasma: quantification of activated Hageman factor-C1 inactivator complexes by an enzyme-linked differential antibody immunosorbent assay. Blood 1985;66:636–41.

51. Atkins PC, Miragliotta G, Talbot SF, et al. Activation of plasma Hageman factor and kallikrein in ongoing allergic reactions in skin. J Immunol 1987;139:2744–8.

52. Wachtfogel YT, Harpel PC, Edmunds LH, et al. Formation of C1s-C1-inhibitor, kallikrein-C1-inhibitor, and plasmin-alpha 2-plasmin-inhibitor complexes during cardiopulmonary bypass. Blood 1989;73:468–71.

53. Nuijens JH, Huijbregts C, Eerenberg-Belmer A, et al. Quantification of plasma factor XIIa-CI-inhibitor and kallikrein-CI-inhibitor complexes in sepsis. Blood 1988;72:1841–8.

54. Malek R, Aulak KS, Davis AE 3rd. The catabolism of intact, reactive centre-cleaved and proteinase-complexed C1 inhibitor in the guinea pig. Clin Exp Immunol 1996;105:191–7.

55. de Smet BJ, de Boer JP, Agterberg J, et al. Clearance of human native, proteinase-complexed, and proteolytically inactivated C1-inhibitor in rats. Blood 1993;81:56–61.

56. Wuillemin WA, Bleeker WK, Agterberg J, et al. Clearance of human factor XIa-inhibitor complexes in rats. Br J Haematol 1996;93:950–4.

57. Perlmutter DH, Glover GI, Rivetna M, et al. Identification of a serpin-enzyme complex receptor on human hepatoma cells and human monocytes. Proc Natl Acad Sci U S A 1990;87:3753–7.

58. van der Linden PW, Struyvenberg A, Kraaijenhagen RJ, et al. Anaphylactic shock after insect-sting challenge in 138 persons with a previous insect-sting reaction. Ann Intern Med 1993;118:161–8.

59. Presanis JS, Hajela K, Ambrus G, et al. Differential substrate and inhibitor profiles for human MASP-1 and MASP-2. Mol Immunol 2004;40:921–9.

60. Kerr FK, Thomas AR, Wijeyewickrema LC, et al. Elucidation of the substrate specificity of the MASP-2 protease of the lectin complement pathway and identification of the enzyme as a major physiological target of the serpin, C1-inhibitor. Mol Immunol 2008;45:670–7.

61. Dobo J, Major B, Kekesi KA, et al. Cleavage of kininogen and subsequent bradykinin release by the complement component: mannose-binding lectin-associated serine protease (MASP)-1. PLoS One 2011;6:e20036.

62. Konings J, Cugno M, Suffritti C, et al. Ongoing contact activation in patients with hereditary angioedema. PLoS One 2013;8:e74043.

63. Esnouf MP, Burgess AI, Dodds AW, et al. A monoclonal antibody raised against human beta-factor XIIa which also recognizes alpha-factor XIIa but not factor XII or complexes of factor XIIa with C1 esterase inhibitor. Thromb Haemost 2000;83:874–81.

64. Papageorgiou PC, Yeo EL, Backx PH, et al. A new enzyme-linked immunosorbent assay recognizing both rat and human activated coagulation factor XII (FXIIa). J Immunol Methods 2012;376:132–8.

65. Nielsen EW, Johansen HT, Hogasen K, et al. Activation of the complement, coagulation, fibrinolytic and kallikrein-kinin systems during attacks of hereditary angioedema. Immunopharmacology 1996;33:359–60.

66. Suffritti C, Zanichelli A, Maggioni L, et al. High-molecular-weight kininogen cleavage correlates with disease states in the bradykinin mediated angioedema due to hereditary c1-inhibitor deficiency. Clin Exp Allergy 2014;44(12):1503–14.

67. Baroso R, Sellier P, Defendi F, et al. Kininogen cleavage assay: diagnostic assistance for kinin-mediated angioedema conditions. PLoS One 2016;11:e0163958.

68. Agostoni A, Cicardi M, Cugno M, et al. Angioedema due to angiotensin-converting enzyme inhibitors. Immunopharmacology 1999;44:21–5.

69. Murphey LJ, Hachey DL, Vaughan DE, et al. Quantification of BK1-5, the stable bradykinin plasma metabolite in humans, by a highly accurate liquid-chromatographic tandem mass spectrometric assay. Anal Biochem 2001;292:87–93.

70. Chen Y, Zhang L, Xu L, et al. Assay of bradykinin metabolites in human body fluids by CE-LIF coupled with transient ITP preconcentration. Electrophoresis 2009;30:2300–6.
71. Joseph K, Tholanikunnel BG, Wolf B, et al. Deficiency of plasminogen activator inhibitor 2 in plasma of patients with hereditary angioedema with normal C1 inhibitor levels. J Allergy Clin Immunol 2016;137(6):1822–9.e1.
72. Csuka D, Veszeli N, Imreh E, et al. Comprehensive study into the activation of the plasma enzyme systems during attacks of hereditary angioedema due to C1-inhibitor deficiency. Orphanet J Rare Dis 2015;10:132.
73. Reshef A, Zanichelli A, Longhurst H, et al. Elevated D-dimers in attacks of hereditary angioedema are not associated with increased thrombotic risk. Allergy 2015; 70:506–13.

Acute Management of Hereditary Angioedema Attacks

Constance H. Katelaris, MD, PhD, FRACP

KEYWORDS

- Hereditary angioedema • HAE acute attacks • Treatment of HAE
- C1-inhibitor concentrate • Icatibant • Ecallantide • rh C1-INH

KEY POINTS

- Management of acute hereditary angioedema (HAE) attacks has changed dramatically over the last decade with 4 clinically proven, options available in some countries.
- Acute treatment options include 2 plasma-derived C1 inhibitor concentrates, a recombinant C1 esterase inhibitor, a kallikrein inhibitor, and a bradykinin 2 receptor antagonist.
- Better education for patients with HAE and adoption of the principles of self-management with "on-demand" treatment have improved quality of life and outcomes for patients.

INTRODUCTION

Modern management of hereditary angioedema (HAE) includes managing the acute attack, short-term prophylaxis for procedures that place the patient at risk of an attack, and long-term management for those where the attack rate is high or impacts adversely on ability to work and conduct daily life.

Acute HAE attack management has changed dramatically over the last 10 years. For more than 2 decades, plasma-derived C1 inhibitor concentrate (pdC1-INH) was the only specific treatment available; now there are 4 clinically proven effective options available, although not all are available in every country as yet. Preferred contemporary use of the treatment options discussed herein is as "on-demand treatment," where treatment is in the hands of the patient to be used once an attack is evident. In this way, delays in treatment access are avoided. Several excellent reviews have explored this topic previously; this article summarizes, in a practical fashion, the

Disclosure Statement: The author has conducted clinical trials with CSL Behring (Berinert) and Shire (icatibant) for which the author have received no personal payments. The author has chaired advisory boards on HAE for Shire Australia and CSL Behring the author has received honoraria for participation in meetings and lectures from Shire Australia and CSL Behring.
Immunology and Allergy Unit, Department of Medicine, Campbelltown Hospital, Therry Road, Campbelltown, Sydney, New South Wales 2560, Australia
E-mail address: Connie.Katelaris@sswahs.nsw.gov.au

attributes of each of these treatment options, listing their indications, risks and bene-fits, and hopefully will serve as a useful guide to those prescribing acute treatment for HAE patients.

MEDICATIONS FOR TREATING ACUTE ATTACKS

Several treatment modalities have become available for management of acute HAE at-tacks in the last 10 to 15 years. Most are now available to patients in North America, Europe, United Kingdom, and Australia, but few of these options exist for many patients living in developing countries.

PLASMA-DERIVED C1 INHIBITOR THERAPY
Berinert

HAE is caused by a deficiency or abnormality in C1-INH, a factor that has numerous inhibitory functions within the contact, fibrinolytic, and complement pathways. Replacement therapy with plasma-derived C1-INH has been used since 1973, with Berinert P first licensed in Germany in 1979. Berinert is nanofiltered and currently licensed for the treatment of acute HAE attacks in Europe, the United States, Australia, and numerous other countries.

Studies of efficacy

A pivotal phase III prospective, multinational, randomized, parallel-group, placebo-controlled, dose-finding, 3-arm, double-blind clinical study (I.M.P.A.C.T. 1 [Interna-tional Multi-center Prospective Angioedema C1-Inhibitor]) assessed the efficacy and safety of Berinert in 124 adult and pediatric patients (6–72 years) who were experi-encing an acute, moderate to severe attack of abdominal or facial HAE.[1] Two doses (10 and 20 U/kg) were compared with placebo, given by intravenous infusion (4 mL/min) within 5 hours of the onset of an attack.

Subjects treated with a 20 U/kg dose experienced a significant reduction ($P = .0025$) in the median time to onset of relief from symptoms of an HAE attack (30 minutes) as compared with placebo (90 minutes). The median time to complete resolution of HAE symptoms was significantly shorter ($P = .0237$) in the Berinert 20 U/kg group (4.9 hours) than in the placebo group (7.8 hours). The study de-monstrated that a 20 U/kg dose of Berinert was significantly more efficacious than 10 U/kg or placebo.

In a subsequent study, Wasserman and colleagues[2] demonstrated that Berinert at 20U/kg dose provided rapid and effective relief for successive abdominal and facial attacks. They treated 663 abdominal attacks in 50 patients and 43 facial attacks in 16 patients. The median time to onset of relief for all attacks was 19.8 minutes, with a median time to complete resolution of 11 hours.

Cinryze

Another pd C1-INH product, Cinryze, is distributed internationally and like Berinert, is purified from human plasma. It was introduced in Europe in 1972 and was approved in 2008 by the Food and Drug Administration in the United States for prophylaxis of HAE.

Zuraw and colleagues[3] reported a randomized trial of nanofiltered C1-INH (Cinryze) for the acute treatment of HAE attacks. Sixty-eight HAE subjects were randomized to receive Cinryze or placebo within 4 hours of the onset of an episode of moderate to severe nonlaryngeal edema (laryngeal episodes were treated with open-label Cinryze). Unlike the Berinert I.M.P.A.C.T. 1 trial, a fixed dose of 1000 U of C1-INH was used in all subjects. There was a significant reduction in time to onset of relief in the treatment group (2 hours) compared with placebo group (>4 hours; P = .02); the proportion of subjects achieving unequivocal relief within 4 hours was 60% (42% in the placebo group; P = .06). Two-thirds of subjects treated with Cinryze required a second dose of the drug at 60 minutes because of inadequate improvement compared with 80% of those treated with placebo. Interestingly, in the open-label extension phase of the trial the rate of response to treatment within 4 hours was 93%; the authors commented on psychological factors affecting perception of pain in abdominal attacks.

Onset of Action of Plasma-Derived C1 Inhibitors

The median times to onset of patient-reported symptom relief were 30 minutes with Berinert 20 U/kg versus 90 minutes with placebo (P = .0025)[1] and 120 minutes with Cinryze 1000 U versus 240 minutes with placebo (P = .02).[4,5]

Rebound and Relapse

In patients with abdominal or facial attacks treated with pd C1-INH 20 U/kg, no new attacks occurred before the complete resolution of the previous attack, indicating an absence of rebound angioedema. Pd C1-INH was generally found to be equally effective and well-tolerated in patients receiving repeated doses.[6]

SPECIFIC CIRCUMSTANCES
Laryngeal Attacks

Approximately 1% of all HAE attacks are laryngeal[7]; 50% of HAE patients will experience a laryngeal attack at some stage. These account for the life-threatening nature of the condition, with death caused by asphyxiation if urgent treatment or airway support is not available. Before effective treatment, 25% to 30% of patients died from a laryngeal attack,[8] with higher numbers (50%) quoted for those with undiagnosed HAE.[9] Studies of patients with untreated laryngeal attacks have demonstrated that an attack may progress over 8 to 24 hours to its peak, persist for 24 to 48 hours and have a mean total duration of 103 hours.[10]

Until recently, data on the efficacy of C1-INH administration in acute laryngeal attacks were limited and empirical,[11] but there trial data are now available to support efficacy.

In an extension of the randomized controlled trial of Berinert, I.M.P.A.C.T 2 enrolled patients in a prospective, open-label study for administration of a single weight-based dose of 20 U/kg of Berinert for treatment of attacks at any location. This study demonstrated the efficacy and safety of the treatment in 16 patients experiencing 39 laryngeal attacks. The median time to onset of relief was 0.25 hours (range, 0.1–1.3) and the median time to complete resolution was 8.25 hours (range, 0.6–48.9). Onset of symptom relief was reported within 1 hour in 95% of patients.[8] There was no evidence of rebound swelling or of diminution in efficacy after repeated administration for other attacks. No emergency procedures such as intubation were required after Berinert treatment. This was also the case in a retrospective case series of 61 patients treated with Berinert for laryngeal attacks reported by Bork and associates.[12] In this, the study mean duration of laryngeal edema in treated patients was 15 hours (208 attacks).

Treatment in Pediatric Patients

There is a lack of systematic studies of acute treatment for HAE attacks in pediatric patients; however, most of the treatments for acute attacks have been used in children and seem to be safe. The use of pdC1-INH for acute attacks of HAE in pediatric patients has been reported in a variety of trials including retrospective cohort studies, prospective open-label studies and randomized placebo-controlled trials.[9,13–15]

Dosing used has varied by product, with fixed dosing for Cinryze and weight-based dosing for Berinert after 2008.

Consensus guidelines recommend use of pdC-1INH in children.[16] In the EU, the United States, and Australia, Berinert is approved for pediatric use. In Europe, Berinert has been used safely in pediatric practice for more than 20 years.[17,18] Cinryze, at a fixed dose of 1000 U, has been used also in pediatric populations.

Craig and colleagues[15] recently reviewed pediatric treatment with pdC1INH in a systematic review, reporting data on nearly 3000 infusions including many in children less than 12 years of age. Children were included in both the Berinert and Cinryze studies, and the results were comparable with those from adult subjects with no adverse effects.

Further evaluation of pediatric data was performed by Lumry and colleagues.[13] Data from 2 randomized, placebo-controlled studies and open-label extensions were analyzed.[3,19,20] Forty-six children and adolescents ranging in age from 2 to 17 years received a total of 2237 Cinryze infusions in the 4 studies. Overall, those receiving active treatment had superior responses. In the open-label extension, 22 children experiencing 121 attacks were evaluated. There were 113 attacks (97%) that had clinical relief within 4 hours after the initial dose of Cinryze. Only 4 attacks (2 gastrointestinal and 2 facial) did not achieve clinical relief within 4 hours.

Pregnancy and Breast Feeding

The safety of pd C1-INH products in pregnancy and lactation has not been proven in controlled clinical trials; however, experience with treatment of women during these periods has not revealed any concerns regarding impact on mother or child. The decision to use Berinert or Cinryze during pregnancy and lactation should be based on clinical need.

ADVERSE EVENTS WITH C1 INHIBITOR PRODUCTS

Berinert has been used for more than 30 years in more than 400,000 treatments and has an excellent safety record.[21] In the pivotal phase III study, the most common adverse effects reported 4 hours after the 20 U/kg dose were nausea, dysgeusia, abdominal pain, and headache; however, no serious adverse events were noted.

Adverse reactions reported with Cinryze have been mild, including nonspecific rash, dizziness, and headaches.

Viral Transmission

Because pd C1-INH is a plasma product, there is the risk of blood-borne viral transmission (**Table 1**). The manufacturing process for Berinert includes pasteurization (at 60°C for 10 hours), hydrophobic interaction chromatography and virus filtration (also called nanofiltration by 2 filters, 20 nm and 15 nm, in series) to reduce the potential for pathogen transmission. In 30 years of postmarketing surveillance, there have been no reports of viral transmission with Berinert.[22]

The manufacturing process used to extract Cinryze from screened human plasma incorporates 3 virus inactivation/removal steps: polyethylene glycol precipitation (20% polyethylene glycol 4000, pH 5.8), pasteurization (10 hours at 60.5 $\pm$ 1.0°C) and 15 nm filtration to remove the smallest known viral particles.

Thromboembolic Events

There have been concerns about thromboembolic events with C1-INH products (see **Table 1**).[23] In postmarketing surveillance of those receiving Berinert for on-demand

Table 1 Specific safety concerns	
Treatment	**Risks**
C1-INH Berinert	Risks associated with blood products, for example, viral transmission (nil recorded in any clinical trial). Very rare reports of thromboembolism.
C1-INH Cinryze	Risks associated with blood products, for example, viral transmission (nil recorded in any clinical trial). Very rare reports of thromboembolism.
RC1-INH Ruconest	Anaphylaxis hypersensitivity to rabbit proteins.
Ecallantide	Hypersensitivity reactions (anaphylaxis).
Icatibant	Injection site reactions.

Abbreviations: C1-INH, C1 inhibitor; RC1-INH, recombinant C1 inhibitor concentrate.

treatment, very few events have been recorded and the majority have been with high-dose off-label use.[24] In the Cinryze studies, the risk of thromboembolic events seemed to be related to prophylactic use, specifically in those with indwelling catheters.

Immunogenicity

Anti-pd C1-INH antibodies were demonstrated in 19% of 57 treated patients but there was no correlation with efficacy or adverse events.[25] Anaphylaxis, although reported, is rare with pdC1-INH.[26,27]

INDICATION AND ADMINISTRATION

Berinert (CSL Behring) is a highly purified, freeze-dried C1-INH derived from human plasma. It contains 500 U of C1-INH per vial (50 U/mL). One unit is equal to the amount of C1-INH in 1 mL of human plasma, which is equivalent to approximately 240 mg/L of plasma. The product is administered intravenously and is immediately available in the plasma, with a plasma concentration corresponding to the administered dose.

Berinert is indicated for the treatment of acute attacks in patients with HAE (Berinert product information; available at: www.cslbehring.com.au).

Cinryze (Shire Pty. Ltd.) is indicated for treatment, preprocedure prophylaxis, and long-term prophylaxis of angioedema in adult and pediatric HAE patients. Recommended treatment dose for an acute episode is 1000 U (2 vials) for adults or children, with provision for a second 1000-U dose after 60 minutes if response is inadequate. Cinryze is supplied as a freeze-dried powder with solvent for reconstitution and can be stored for up to 2 years at room temperature (<25°C). After reconstitution, a single dose is 1000 U/10 mL with a concentration of 100 U/mL. Regulatory labeling in Europe and the United States allows self-administration of both plasma C1INH products with appropriate patient education and training (**Table 2**).

RECOMBINANT C1 INHIBITOR CONESTAT ALFA

A brief review of the data on recombinant C1-INH (rh C1-INH) is given. More detailed information has been provided in a recent review.[28]

Introduction

Conestat alfa is a human recombinant C1 esterase inhibitor (rh C1-INH), developed as an alternative to pd C1-INH, to address the potential risks of bloodborne pathogen transmission that exists with plasma-derived products. It has a sequence identical

Table 2
Dosing

Treatment	Dosing to Treat HAE Attack	Product Details
Pd C1-INH (Berinert)	20 U/kg, slow IV administration, 4 mL/min; with appropriate training, suitable for home/self-administration.	Highly purified, freeze-dried C1-INH derived from human plasma. It contains 500 U of C1-INH per vial (50 U/mL). Supplied as 1 carton containing the single-use vial of Berinert and one 10-mL vial of water for injection, and a second carton containing 1 Mix2Vial filter transfer set, a disposable 10-mL syringe, an infusion set, 2 alcohol swabs, and a plaster (adhesive bandage). Store below 25°C.
Pd C1-INH (Cinryze)	1000 U (2 vials) for adults or children, with provision for a second 1000-U dose after 60 minutes if response is inadequate. IV administration; with appropriate training suitable for home/self-administration.	Single-use vial of glass containing 500 U of C1 esterase inhibitor as a nanofiltered, freeze-dried powder. The vial is sealed with a rubber type I stopper, and an aluminum seal with a plastic flip-off cap. *Solvent*: 5 mL of water for injections in a vial of colorless glass, which is closed with a rubber stopper and an aluminum seal with a plastic flip off cap.
Rh C1-INH (Ruconest)	50 IU/kg for patients weighing <84 kg; up to 4200 IU for patients weighing ≥84 kg; administered as a slow IV injection over 5 min. An additional dose of the same recommended amount can be administered if symptoms persist, but do not exceed 2 doses in 24 h; with appropriate training suitable for home/self-administration.	Lyophilized powder for reconstitution for injection in a single-use 25-mL glass vial containing 2100 IU of rhC1INH per vial
Ecallantide	30 mg (3 vials per dose) subcutaneously; given by a health care provider.	Clear solution, three 10 mg/mL single-use vials packaged in a carton. Each vial contains 10 mg of ecallantide. Keep refrigerated (2°C–8°C/36°F–46°F). Vials removed from refrigeration should be stored below 86°F/30°C and used within 14 d or returned to refrigeration until use.
Icatibant	30 mg injected subcutaneously in the abdominal area. If response is inadequate or symptoms recur, additional injections of 30 mg may be administered at intervals of ≥6 h. Do not administer >3 injections in 24 h. Patients may self-administer upon recognition of an HAE attack.	Pre-filled syringe, 30 mg/3 mL.
FFP	Two units of FFP are given, repeating 2–4 hourly until there is benefit. Administered in health care facility.	

Abbreviations: C1-INH, C1 inhibitor; FFP, fresh frozen plasma; HAE, hereditary angioedema; Pd C1-INH, plasma-derived C1 inhibitor concentrate; RC1-INH, recombinant C1 inhibitor concentrate.

to the natural protein so it has an identical mode of action to human C1-INH. There are differences in the glycosylation of rh C1-INH and pdC1-INH that do not affect rh C1-INH specificity, but result in a shorter half-life compared with pd C1-INH.[29]

Recombinant human C1-INH is purified from the milk of genetically modified rabbits.[30] The benefit of recombinant technology is that it enables a reliable supply of a product with uniform quality. One international unit of rh C1INH activity is defined as the equivalent of C1 esterase inhibiting activity present in 1 mL of pooled normal plasma. Population pharmacokinetic modeling supports a dosing scheme of 50 IU/kg, which achieves C1INH levels above the lower level of the normal range (0.7 U/mL) in at least 94% of patients.[31]

Trial Data

The efficacy of rh C1-INH in the treatment of acute attacks in HAE patients has been evaluated in 3 randomized, double-blind, placebo-controlled studies [32–34] and 3 open-label extension studies[35–38] using patient-reported outcomes with a validated visual analog scale instrument. The North American study used rh C1-INH at 50 and 100 IU/kg, demonstrating effectiveness and safety of both doses, while the European study used a dose of 100 IU/kg showing similar superiority over placebo.[32] The treatment was effective for HAE attacks at various sites.

Open-label extension studies[35,36] demonstrated that efficacy was maintained for subsequent acute HAE attacks. In these 2 studies, 362 attacks in 119 patients were treated with 80% of repeat attacks responding within 4 hours and most requiring only a single dose of rh C1-INH.

Li and colleagues[37] conducted an open-label extension study evaluating the efficacy and safety of the treatment of multiple HAE attacks in North American and European patients. For 44 patients experiencing 224 HAE attacks, a single 50 IU/kg dose of rh C1-INH was effective for improving symptoms of an HAE attack and the incidence of symptom relapse was low for initial and subsequent attacks. Almost all attacks were treated with only a single dose of rh C1-INH. A total of 215 of 224 attacks (96%) were treated with a single 50-IU/kg dose of rh C1-INH, and no increase in dose was needed for treatments of repeat attacks.

Onset of Action

In the pivotal trials, patients were treated within 5 hours of onset of HAE attack symptoms. The primary efficacy endpoint was the median time to onset of symptom relief. A pooled analysis indicated a significantly faster onset of symptom relief for both doses of rh C1-INH, 50 U/kg (122 minutes; 95% confidence interval, 72–136; $P = .013$) and 100 U/kg (66 minutes; 95% confidence interval, 61–122; $P = .001$), versus placebo (495 minutes; 95% confidence interval, 245–520).[28,32]

Rebound and Relapse

In the study by Li and colleagues,[37] the vast majority (96%) of patients required only 1 dose of rh C1-INH. Relapse within 24 hours of treatment for patients responding to a single dose of rh C-1INH has been low in all clinical trials to date.[32,36]

Response by Anatomic Location

In the North American open-label study,[36] the median time to onset of relief at different anatomic locations (most attacks were peripheral or abdominal) with both doses of rh C1-INH (range, 50–124 minutes) was faster than with placebo (range, 243–560 minutes). Few attacks (10%) required treatment with a second dose, and of these, most were orofacial or pharyngeal–laryngeal attacks.

In the European open-label study, the fastest median time to symptomatic relief occurred with abdominal attacks (33 minutes), followed by peripheral attacks (61 minutes), orofacial and pharyngeal–laryngeal attacks (120 minutes), and genitourinary attacks (480 minutes).[35]

SPECIAL POPULATIONS
Pediatric Use

The safety and efficacy of rh C1-INH was evaluated in 17 adolescent patients (13–17 years of age) treated for 52 HAE attacks. No serious adverse reactions were reported in these patients, with the most common reactions being abdominal pain, headache, and oropharyngeal pain.

Pregnancy and Breast Feeding

Rh C1-INH is pregnancy category B. There are, however, no adequate and well-controlled studies in pregnant women. It should only be used during pregnancy if clearly needed. It is not known if rh C1-INH is excreted in human milk.[30]

Adverse Events

Rh C1-INH is contraindicated in patients with a history of allergy to rabbits or rabbit-derived products and in patients with a history of life-threatening immediate hypersensitivity reactions, including anaphylaxis, to C1 esterase inhibitor preparations (see **Table 1**).[29] Anaphylaxis was the most serious adverse reaction during the clinical studies of rh C1-INH; headache, nausea, and diarrhea were the most common adverse reactions ($\geq$2%) with a similar incidence to that reported with placebo.

Immunogenicity
Preexposure and postexposure testing of patients in all the trials demonstrated a very low potential for induction of anti-drug–related or anti–host–related antibodies.[28]

Thrombogenicity
To date, there have been no signals from the various trials that there is a risk of thromboembolic complications.[39]

Administration

Ruconest is supplied in 25-mL vials containing 2100 IU rh C1INH for reconstitution with sterile water for injection. It is administered using weight-based dosing of 50 IU/kg as a slow IV injection over 5 minutes and may be self-administered by the patient after appropriate training (see **Table 2**).

ECALLANTIDE
Introduction

Ecallantide (Kalbitor Dyax Corp) is a 60-amino acid recombinant protein discovered through phage display technology. A potent kallikrein inhibitor, it blocks the plasma-binding site resulting in reduced bradykinin production. Kallikrein plays a role in the activation of factor XIIa and that function is also blocked by ecallantide.

The absolute bioavailability of ecallantide is approximately 90%; sex, age, and body weight do not significantly affect exposure. Its metabolism is not via cytochrome P-450 isoenzyme pathways, so drug interactions via these isoenzymes are not expected. It is eliminated by the kidneys.

Clinical Trial Data

The efficacy and dosage for ecallantide were studied in 3 phase II and 2 phase III trials known as the EDEMA trials (Evaluation of DX-88's Effect in Mitigating Angioedema). EDEMA 3 and EDEMA 4 had similar designs as randomized, double-blind, placebo-controlled studies enrolling adolescents and adults, using the treatment outcome score and the mean symptom complex severity score as endpoints. Both studies had open-label extension phases. A total of 168 patients were enrolled across the 2 studies. The results from these trials demonstrated that ecallantide is an effective treatment for acute attacks of HAE and acts by both preventing progression and reducing HAE symptoms. In addition to the individual results from EDEMA 3 and EDEMA 4, integrated analysis of the 2 trials further illustrated the effectiveness of ecallantide in relieving acute HAE attacks.[40–42]

Onset of Action

MacGinnitie and colleagues,[43] analyzing results from EDEMA 3 and 4, demonstrated the onset of action of ecallantide to be within 4 hours with median time to improvement of 2 hours. These figures resemble those published for C1-INH (range, 2.0–2.9 hours) and icatibant (range, 2.0–2.5 hours).

Rebound

Bernstein and colleagues[44] performed a post hoc analysis of EDEMA3 and 4 to investigate the likelihood of relapse or rebound symptoms after ecallantide treatment. One of 42 patients treated with ecallantide included in analysis, demonstrated likely relapse (2.4%), with an additional 3 patients showing possible relapse or rebound (7.2%). Pooled clinical trial data revealed that 12% of ecallantide-treated patients received a second ecallantide dose and this need was associated with the occurrence of peripheral attacks. There was no increase in treatment-related adverse events with a second dose of ecallantide.[45]

Laryngeal Attacks

Treatment response to ecallantide has been shown to be related to anatomic site of the attack, with abdominal and laryngeal attacks responding better than attacks involving peripheral sites.[46] The efficacy of ecallantide for treating laryngeal attacks has been studied specifically by Sheffer.[47] The investigator analyzed 4 clinical studies (EDEMA2, EDEMA3, EDEMA4, and DX-88/19) that included 98 patients treated with ecallantide 30 mg subcutaneously for 220 laryngeal attacks. Eighty percent of patients experienced sustained improvement after ecallantide treatment and 63% achieved complete or near-complete resolution of symptoms within 4 hours of dosing.

Special Populations

The Food and Drug Administration extended approval of ecallantide use to 12 years and older in 2014.

Ecallantide is a pregnancy category C as assigned by the Food and Drug Administration because animal studies demonstrated developmental toxicity. The use of ecallantide in breastfeeding women is cautioned against because it is not known whether ecallantide is excreted in breast milk and it is not known what effects it may have on a developing, growing infant (Kalbitor prescribing info revised March 2015; available at: http://www.kalbitor.com/hcp/rems/pdf/KalbitorFullPrescribing- Information.pdf).

Adverse Events

In the patients enrolled in EDEMA 3 and 4, treatment-related side effects were reported in 11.1% of patients receiving study drug compared with 13.9% in those receiving placebo. Headache, nausea, fatigue, diarrhea, upper respiratory tract infection, injection site reactions, nasopharyngitis, vomiting, pruritus, abdominal pain, and pyrexia were the most common complaints.

Anaphylaxis

Anaphylaxis occurred in 4% of HAE patients treated with ecallantide.[48,49] For this reason, ecallantide is only approved for administration by a health care professional in a setting with appropriate medical support (see **Table 1**).

Immunogenicity

There is a risk of antibody formation to ecallantide and this was found in nearly 5% of patients; however, the significance of this is unknown. There seems to be no correlation between antibody formation and anaphylaxis in patients receiving ecallantide nor did antibody formation affect clinical efficacy.[48]

Administration

The drug concentration of each vial of ecallantide is 10 mg/mL; the recommended dose of ecallantide is 30 mg given as three 10-mg subcutaneous injections. The formulation should be kept refrigerated and protected from light. Once removed from the refrigerator, the drug is stable for 14 days (see **Table 2**). Ecallantide is approved for administration by a health care professional in a setting with appropriate medical support. (Kalbitor prescribing info revised March 2015; available at: http://www.kalbitor.com/hcp/rems/pdf/KalbitorFullPrescribing- Information.pdf).

ICATIBANT
Introduction

A major mediator of swelling in HAE is bradykinin, exerting its effects via the B2 receptor expressed on vascular endothelium. Binding leads to generation of numerous inflammatory mediators resulting in vasodilatation and edema. Icatibant, as a potent B2 receptor antagonist, has proven to be a specific and effective treatment for HAE attacks Icatibant is a synthetic decapeptide with a similar structure to bradykinin. It has an excellent bioavailability profile when given subcutaneously, with rapid absorption from the injection site and peak concentrations reached within 30 minutes. It has a terminal half-life of 1 to 2 hours and undergoes hepatic metabolism before renal excretion. Cytochrome P450 enzymes are not involved in the metabolism of icatibant and dose adjustments are not needed in renal and hepatic impairment, although clearance is reduced in old age. It does cross the placenta and in rodent studies was shown to be excreted in breast milk. An open-label study in 15 patients established the dose of 30 mg as optimal.[50]

Studies of Efficacy

The efficacy and safety of icatibant have been evaluated in 3 double-blind, randomized, controlled trials known as FAST (For Angioedema Subcutaneous Treatment) 1, 2, and 3.[51,52] FAST 2 compared icatibant with tranexamic acid, whereas FAST 1 and 3 were placebo controlled. The inclusion criteria for all 3 FAST studies were individuals, greater than 18 years of age, diagnosed with HAE 1 or 2. Pregnant and lactating women were excluded from the studies.

The FAST-1 trial compared subcutaneous injection of icatibant with placebo in 57 subjects presenting acutely with superficial cutaneous or abdominal angioedema episodes. The primary outcome measure was the time to onset of a 30% symptom improvement, but unfortunately the results for the combined group did not attain statistical significance. This result was attributed to the placebo arm having a higher use of rescue medication including C1-INH increasing the overall perceived effectiveness of the placebo arm.

The FAST-2 trial compared subcutaneous icatibant with oral tranexamic acid using a double-blind, double-dummy design. In this trial, the median time to onset, 30% improvement, and almost complete symptom relief was significantly better in the icatibant group (0.8, 2.0, and 10.0 hours, respectively) than in the tranexamic acid group (7.9, 12.0, and 51.0 hours, respectively).

FAST 3 was a further placebo-controlled, randomized, double-blind trial in 88 subjects with HAE presenting with acute episodes affecting the abdomen, periphery, or airway. The primary endpoint of 50% reduction in symptom scores was significantly different between active treatment (2.0 hours) and placebo (19.8 hours). The time to initial symptom relief was 0.8 hours versus 3.5 hours.

Laryngeal Attacks

Eight patients in FAST 1 and 3 patients in FAST 2 received open-label icatibant for laryngeal attacks and the time to symptom improvement was 0.6 hours and 1.0 hour, respectively. At 4 hours after icatibant administration, 9 of the 11 patients were symptom free and the remaining 2 had mild symptoms.[51] In the FAST 3 trial, a total of 21 subjects with 21 laryngeal attacks received icatibant. The median time to 50% or more reduction in symptom severity was 2.5 hours with icatibant versus 3.2 hours with placebo.[52]

In a further analysis, Lumry and colleagues[53] reported trial data to evaluate the efficacy and safety of icatibant for the repeated treatment of multiple HAE attacks at any location including laryngeal attacks. In groups of patients with 1 to 5 icatibant-treated attacks at any location (n = 88), the median times to onset of symptom relief, onset of primary symptom relief and almost complete symptom relief were 1.9 to 2.1, 1.5 to 2.0, and 3.5 to 19.7 hours, respectively. The same outcomes for laryngeal attacks (n = 25) were 1.0 to 2.0, 1.0 to 2.0, and 1.5 to 8.1 hours, respectively. The analyses supported the sustained efficacy and safety profile of icatibant when used to treat multiple HAE attacks at any location, including laryngeal.

Adverse Events

Injection site reactions are the most common reported side effect after icatibant injection (see **Table 1**). Otherwise, its side effect profile across a number of studies was no different to that of placebo. Animal studies have demonstrated that blocking the B2 receptor can affect coronary blood flow adversely, so acute cardiac or cerebral ischemia and unstable angina are relative contraindications to its use.

Indications and Administration

Icatibant is supplied as a prefilled syringe, 30 mg/3 mL and has a shelf life of 2 years if stored at 4°C (see **Table 2**). Currently, it is indicated for the acute treatment of HAE attacks in those 18 years of age and older; however, trials in pediatric populations are underway.

Self-Administration

A large, prospective, open-label phase IIIb (EASSI [Evaluation of the Safety of Self-administration with Icatibant]) study has been conducted to evaluate the safety of self-administration injections. Overall, self-administration of icatibant for an acute attack of HAE was shown to be safe and effective in the 56 patients evaluated[54] and icatibant is licensed for patient self-administration.

Other Considerations

Lack of efficacy of tranexamic acid for acute hereditary angioedema attacks

Any consideration that tranexamic acid may be used to treat acute HAE attacks has been removed by the demonstration of lack of efficacy in the FAST 3 trial where it was used as a comparator for icatibant.[52,55]

FRESH FROZEN PLASMA

In many parts of the world, FFP is the only available treatment for acute HAE attacks. For years, FFP, which contains C1-INH, has been used in treatment of acute attacks of HAE, but there may be worsening of symptoms because of enhanced consumption of C1-INH by substrate proteins. No controlled studies have been conducted investigating its role or efficacy. It involves risks of transmissible infectious disease caused by nonpasteurized fresh frozen plasma products and transfusion reactions. When used, 2 U of FFP are given, repeating after 2 to 4 hours until there is benefit (see **Table 2**).[56]

Preparedness to Intubate

There are now a number of options for the acute treatment of upper airway edema in HAE. Patients need careful education about the early signs and symptoms of upper airway involvement and the need for prompt administration of their medical therapy. It is essential that, if upper airway swelling occurs, they present as soon as possible to a medical a facility where intensive care management is available and they can be observed until complete resolution of symptoms. If alarming signs of airway obstruction (such as stridor, dyspnea, and signs of respiratory arrest) occur, airway patency should be reestablished and oxygen administered. If stridor, hoarseness, or hypoxemia are present, immediate intubation is essential. The severity of the edema may interfere with endotracheal intubation, requiring airway patency be restored by surgical intervention when intubation is not feasible.[57]

Patient Self-Administration

Recent consensus guidelines emphasize the importance of patients having prompt access to therapies for management of acute attacks known as "on-demand therapy."[16,58–60] In this model of care, patients are trained to self-administer treatment either by subcutaneous injection for icatibant or by intravenous infusion for C1 inhibitor concentrate. This allows early treatment of attacks and limits the time of disability and discomfort caused by an attack as well as preventing complications resulting from progression to severe angioedema symptoms.

SUMMARY

Over the last decade, the development of new treatments and demonstration of their efficacy in placebo-controlled clinical trials have dramatically improved the outlook for patients with HAE. Recognition of the importance of comprehensive education and training in self-management have created the opportunity for autonomy and prompt treatment for many patients with HAE, thereby reducing greatly the impact of this distressing condition on daily life.[58]

Unfortunately, effective and timely management of HAE attacks is not an option for those who live in developing countries, where these drugs are not available. All the agents discussed are high-cost drugs and their availability is limited in many parts of the world. Our challenge is to find mechanisms by which effective treatment may be made available to all who have a diagnosis of HAE. There is still much to learn about the best and most cost-effective management strategies for the individual patient with HAE. Ultimately, we look forward to a time when acute management of attacks is not necessary as new agents are developed with the capacity to restore homeostasis and completely prevent occurrence of angioedema attacks.

REFERENCES

1. Bernstein JA, Levy R, Wasserman RL, et al. Treatment of acute abdominal and facial attacks of hereditary angioedema (HAE) with human C1 esterase inhibitor (C1-INH): results of a global, multicenter, randomized, placebo-controlled, phase II/III study (I.M.P.A.C.T.1). J Allergy Clin Immunol 2008;121(3):795.
2. Wasserman RL, Levy RJ, Bewtra AK, et al. Prospective study of C1 esterase inhibitor in the treatment of successive acute abdominal and facial hereditary angioedema attacks. Ann Allergy Asthma Immunol 2011;106(1):62–8.
3. Zuraw BL, Busse PJ, White M, et al. Nanofiltered C1 inhibitor concentrate for treatment of hereditary angioedema. N Engl J Med 2010;363(6):513–22.
4. Riedl MA. Update on the acute treatment of hereditary angioedema. Allergy Asthma Proc 2011;32(1):11–6.
5. Bhardwaj N, Craig TJ. Treatment of hereditary angioedema: a review (CME). Transfusion 2014;54(11):2989–96.
6. Bork K. Current management options for hereditary angioedema. Curr Allergy Asthma Rep 2012;12(4):273–80.
7. Lang DM, Aberer W, Bernstein JA, et al. International consensus on hereditary and acquired angioedema. Ann Allergy Asthma Immunol 2012;109(6):395–402.
8. Craig TJ, Wasserman RL, Levy RJ, et al. Prospective study of rapid relief provided by C1 esterase inhibitor in emergency treatment of acute laryngeal attacks in hereditary angioedema. J Clin Immunol 2010;30(6):823–9.
9. Craig TJ, Levy RJ, Wasserman RL, et al. Efficacy of human C1 esterase inhibitor concentrate compared with placebo in acute hereditary angioedema attacks. J Allergy Clin Immunol 2009;124(4):801–8.
10. Christiansen SC, Zuraw BL. Hereditary angioedema: management of laryngeal attacks. Am J Rhinol Allergy 2011;25(6):379–82.
11. Farkas H, Harmat G, Füst G, et al. Clinical management of hereditary angioedema in children. Pediatr Allergy Immunol 2002;13(3):153–61.
12. Bork K, Hardt J, Schicketanz K-H, et al. Clinical studies of sudden upper airway obstruction in patients with hereditary angioedema due to C1 esterase inhibitor deficiency. Arch Intern Med 2003;163(10):1229–35.
13. Lumry W, Manning ME, Hurewitz DS, et al. Nanofiltered C1-esterase inhibitor for the acute management and prevention of hereditary angioedema attacks due to C1-inhibitor deficiency in children. J Pediatr 2013;162(5):1017–22.e1–2.
14. Schneider L, Hurewitz D, Wasserman R, et al. C1-INH concentrate for treatment of acute hereditary angioedema: a pediatric cohort from the I.M.P.A.C.T. studies. Pediatr Allergy Immunol 2013;24(1):54–60.
15. Craig TJ, Schneider LC, MacGinnitie AJ. Plasma-derived C1-INH for managing hereditary angioedema in pediatric patients: a systematic review. Pediatr Allergy Immunol 2015;26(6):537–44.

16. Craig T. WAO Guidelines for the management of hereditary angioedema. WAO Journal 2012;5:182–99.
17. Farkas H. Pediatric hereditary angioedema due to C1-inhibitor deficiency. Allergy Asthma Clin Immunol 2010;6(1):18–28.
18. Wahn V, Aberer W, Eberl W, et al. Hereditary angioedema (HAE) in children and adolescents–a consensus on therapeutic strategies. Eur J Pediatr 2012;171(9): 1339–48.
19. Riedl MA, Hurewitz DS, Levy R, et al. Nanofiltered C1 esterase inhibitor (human) for the treatment of acute attacks of hereditary angioedema: an open-label trial. Ann Allergy Asthma Immunol 2012;108(1):49–53.
20. Zuraw BL, Kalfus I. Safety and efficacy of prophylactic nanofiltered C1-inhibitor in hereditary angioedema. Am J Med 2012;125(9):938.e1-7.
21. Bork K, Steffense I, Neme A, et al. A systematic review of the efficacy and safety of a purified, pasteurized C1 inhibitor concentrate for the treatment of patients with type I or II hereditary angioedema. Allergy Asthma Clin Immunol 2010; 6(Suppl 1):P32.
22. De Serres J, Gruter A, Linder J. Safety and efficacy of pasteurized C1 inhibitor concentrate (Berinert P)in hereditary angioedema: a review. Transfus Apher Sci 2013;29(3):247–54.
23. Bork K. Pasteurized and nanofiltered, plasma-derived C1 esterase inhibitor concentrate for the treatment of hereditary angioedema. Immunotherapy 2014; 6(5):533–51.
24. Zanichelli A, Wu MA, Andreoli A, et al. The safety of treatments for angioedema with hereditary C1 inhibitor deficiency. Expert Opin Drug Saf 2015;14(11): 1725–36.
25. Craig TJ, Bewtra AK, Hurewitz D, et al. Treatment response after repeated administration of C1 esterase inhibitor for successive acute hereditary angioedema attacks. Allergy Asthma Proc 2012;33(4):354–61.
26. Cicardi M, Zingale LC, Zanichelli A. A patient with hereditary angioedema who experienced anaphylaxis in response to C1 esterase inhibitor is successfully treated with DX-88 (Ecallantide), a potent human kallikrein inhibitor: a case study. Mol Immunol 2007;44:160–1.
27. Riedl MA, Bygum A, Lumry W, et al, Berinert Registry Investigators. Safety and usage of C1-inhibitor in hereditary angioedema: berinert registry data. J Allergy Clin Immunol Pract 2016;4(5):963–71.
28. Riedl M. Recombinant human C1 esterase inhibitor in the management of hereditary angioedema. Clin Drug Investig 2015;35(7):407–17.
29. Ruconest prescribing information. Available at: https://www.ruconest.com/hcp/. Accessed January 10, 2016.
30. Cruz MP. Conestat Alfa (Ruconest). Pharm Ther 2015;40(2):109–14.
31. Farrell C, Hayes S, Relan A, et al. Population pharmacokinetics of recombinant human C1 inhibitor in patients with hereditary angioedema. Br J Clin Pharmacol 2013;76(6):897–907.
32. Zuraw B, Cicardi M, Levy RJ, et al. Recombinant human C1-inhibitor for the treatment of acute angioedema attacks in patients with hereditary angioedema. J Allergy Clin Immunol 2010;126(4):821–7.e14.
33. Riedl MA, Bernstein JA, Li H, et al. Recombinant human C1-esterase inhibitor relieves symptoms of hereditary angioedema attacks: phase 3, randomized, placebo-controlled trial. Ann Allergy Asthma Immunol 2014;112(2):163–9.e1.

34. Reshef A, Moldovan D, Obtulowicz K, et al. Recombinant human C1 inhibitor for the prophylaxis of hereditary angioedema attacks: a pilot study. Allergy 2012; 68(1):118–24.

35. Moldovan D, Reshef A, Fabiani J, et al. Efficacy and safety of recombinant human C1-inhibitor for the treatment of attacks of hereditary angioedema: European open-label extension study. Clin Exp Allergy 2012;42(6):929–35.

36. Riedl MA, Levy RJ, Suez D, et al. Efficacy and safety of recombinant C1 inhibitor for the treatment of hereditary angioedema attacks: a North American open-label study. Ann Allergy Asthma Immunol 2013;110(4):295–9.

37. Li HH, Moldovan D, Bernstein JA, et al. Recombinant human-C1 inhibitor is effective and safe for repeat hereditary angioedema attacks. J Allergy Clin Immunol Pract 2015;3(3):417–23.

38. Caliezi C, Wuillemin WA, Zeerleder S, et al. C1-Esterase inhibitor: an anti-inflammatory agent and its potential use in the treatment of diseases other than hereditary angioedema. Pharmacol Rev 2000;52(1):91–112.

39. Relan A, Bakhtiari K, van Amersfoort ES, et al. Recombinant C1-inhibitor: effects on coagulation and fibrinolysis in patients with hereditary angioedema. BioDrugs 2012;26(1):43–52.

40. Levy RJ, Lumry WR, McNeil DL, et al. EDEMA4: a phase 3, double-blind study of subcutaneous ecallantide treatment for acute attacks of hereditary angioedema. Ann Allergy Asthma Immunol 2010;104(6):523–9.

41. Cicardi M, Levy RJ, McNeil DL, et al. Ecallantide for the treatment of acute attacks in hereditary angioedema. N Engl J Med 2010;363(6):523–31.

42. Sheffer AL, Campion M, Levy RJ, et al. Ecallantide (DX-88) for acute hereditary angioedema attacks: integrated analysis of 2 double-blind, phase 3 studies. J Allergy Clin Immunol 2011;128(1):153–4.

43. MacGinnitie AJ, Campion M, Stolz LE, et al. Ecallantide for treatment of acute hereditary angioedema attacks: analysis of efficacy by patient characteristics. Allergy Asthma Proc 2012;33(2):178–85.

44. Bernstein JA, Shea EP, Koester J, et al. Assessment of rebound and relapse following ecallantide treatment for acute attacks of hereditary angioedema. Allergy 2012;67(9):1173–80.

45. Li HH, Campion M, Craig TJ, et al. Analysis of hereditary angioedema attacks requiring a second dose of ecallantide. Ann Allergy Asthma Immunol 2013; 110(3):168–72.

46. Bernstein JA, Qazi M. Ecallantide: its pharmacology, pharmacokinetics, clinical efficacy and tolerability. Expert Rev Clin Immunol 2010;6(1):29–39.

47. Sheffer AL. Hereditary angioedema: optimal therapy. J Allergy Clin Immunol 2007;120(4):756–7.

48. Garnock-Jones KP. Ecallantide in acute hereditary angioedema: profile report. BioDrugs 2011;25(1):51–3.

49. Craig TJ, Li HH, Riedl M, et al. Characterization of anaphylaxis after ecallantide treatment of hereditary angioedema attacks. J Allergy Clin Immunol Pract 2015;3(2):206–12.e4.

50. Bork K, Frank J, Grundt B, et al. Treatment of acute edema attacks in hereditary angioedema with a bradykinin receptor-2 antagonist (Icatibant). J Allergy Clin Immunol 2007;119(6):1497–503.

51. Cicardi M, Banerji A, Bracho F, et al. Icatibant, a new bradykinin-receptor antagonist, in hereditary angioedema. N Engl J Med 2010;363(6):532–41.

52. Lumry WR, Li HH, Levy RJ, et al. Randomized placebo-controlled trial of the bradykinin B_2 receptor antagonist icatibant for the treatment of acute attacks of

hereditary angioedema: the FAST-3 trial. Ann Allergy Asthma Immunol 2011; 107(6):529–37.

53. Lumry WR, Farkas H, Moldovan D, et al. Icatibant for multiple hereditary angioedema attacks across the controlled and open-label extension phases of FAST-3. Int Arch Allergy Immunol 2015;168(1):44–55.

54. Ghazi A, Grant JA. Hereditary angioedema: epidemiology, management, and role of icatibant. Biologics 2013;7:103–11.

55. Longhurst HJ. Management of acute attacks of hereditary angioedema: potential role of icatibant. Vasc Health Risk Manag 2010;6:795–802.

56. Longhurst HJ. Emergency treatment of acute attacks in hereditary angioedema due to C1 inhibitor deficiency: what is the evidence? Int J Clin Pract 2005; 59(5):594–9.

57. Farkas H. Management of upper airway edema caused by hereditary angioedema. Allergy Asthma Clin Immunol 2010;6(1):19–27.

58. Zanichelli A, Mansi M, Azin GM, et al. Efficacy of on-demand treatment in reducing morbidity in patients with hereditary angioedema due to C1 inhibitor deficiency. Allergy 2015;70(12):1553–8.

59. Zuraw BL, Bernstein JA, Lang DM. A focused parameter update: hereditary angioedema, acquired C1 inhibitor deficiency, and angiotensin-converting enzyme inhibitor–associated angioedema. J Allergy Clin Immunol 2013;131:1491–3.e25.

60. Cicardi M, Bork K, Caballero T, et al. Evidence-based recommendations for the therapeutic management of angioedema owing to hereditary C1 inhibitor deficiency: consensus report of an International Working Group. Allergy 2012;67(2): 147–57.

Prophylactic Therapy for Hereditary Angioedema

Hilary Longhurst, MA, FRCP, PhD, FRCPath*, Emily Zinser, MA, MBBS, MRCP

KEYWORDS

- Prophylaxis • Hereditary angioedema • Androgens • Tranexamic acid
- Progestagens • C1 inhibitor

KEY POINTS

- Androgens are effective prophylactic agents in many patients with hereditary angioedema but are limited by their side effect profile.
- C1 inhibitor has a more favorable tolerability profile but requires intravenous delivery at current licensing and may require dose titration for maximum efficacy.
- Progestagens and tranexamic acid may have a role as prophylaxis; efficacy is inferior to that of androgens but their favorable side effect profiles make them potential options for women and children.
- Short-term prophylaxis should be considered for all procedures, with most evidence for efficacy of C1 inhibitor concentrate.

INTRODUCTION

Given the social, psychological, and financial implications of recurrent angioedema, effective prophylaxis has significant potential in improving attack frequency and severity, and subsequent quality of life.

The aim of prophylaxis is to reduce and, ideally, prevent attacks of angioedema. Interventions therefore are potentially lifelong, while hereditary angioedema (HAE) remains treatable but incurable. Prophylaxis therefore needs to be considered alongside comorbidities, drug interactions, side effects, and patient preference, and may need to be changed as these parameters alter throughout life. Prophylaxis also

Disclosure: Dr H. Longhurst is a medical advisor to HAEUK. She and members of her department have received funding to attend conferences and other educational events, have acted as medical advisor or speaker, have received donations to her departmental fund, have received financial and other assistance with patient care projects, and/or have participated in clinical trials with the following companies: Biocryst, CSL Behring and Shire. Dr E. Zinser has no conflicts of interest.

Department of Immunology, Barts Health NHS Trust, Pathology and Pharmacy Building, 80 Newark Street, London E1 2HS, UK
* Corresponding author.
E-mail address: Hilary.longhurst@bartshealth.nhs.uk

needs to be considered in the context of patient individual factors, including location of nearest emergency department facilities, ease of intravenous (IV) access, and frequency and location of attacks.

WHEN PROPHYLAXIS IS INDICATED

Different guidelines take different approaches to prophylaxis, as outlined in **Table 1**. Prophylaxis does not guarantee elimination of attacks, so reinforcement of an up-to-date and effective acute attack plan is of paramount importance. Importantly, previous attack patterns, including absence of laryngeal edema, do not necessarily reflect future course.[5]

ATTENUATED ANDROGENS
Efficacy

Early placebo-controlled trials involved small numbers of patients but showed a beneficial effect; in one randomized, double-blind, placebo-controlled trial, 9 patients were treated with either placebo or 200 mg of danazol 3 times a day until 28 days elapsed or an HAE attack occurred, at which point patients crossed over to the other treatment arm. Attacks occurred in 93.6% of placebo courses but 2.2% of danazol courses (P<.001).[6] Another randomized trial assessed 10 mg/d methyltestosterone versus placebo in 4 male patients, with crossover after an attack or 3 months of treatment. After 11.8 months, placebo administration was completed, with 19 attacks, compared with 46 months of androgen therapy, with 4 attacks (P<.001).[7] Furthermore, laryngeal

Table 1 Recent guidelines on indications for long-term prophylaxis in hereditary Angioedema		
Guidelines Source	**Year Published**	**Indications for Long-Term Prophylaxis**
Canadian Hereditary Angioedema Guidelines[1]	2014	• On-demand treatment alone does not allow patients to lead healthy and productive lives • Suboptimal efficacy of on-demand treatment to control attack severity and frequency • Also consider: frequency and severity of previous attacks, access to emergency treatment, ability to administer on-demand therapy
World Allergy Organization[2]	2012	• All severely symptomatic patients • Also consider disease severity, attack frequency, quality of life, availability of resources, and failure to achieve control with on-demand therapy
US Hereditary Angioedema Association Medical Advisory Board[3]	2013	• Consider attack frequency and severity, co-morbidities, access to emergency treatment, patient experience and preference
Hereditary Angioedema International Working Group (HAWK)[4]	2012	Majority opinion: long-term prophylaxis indicated if, in the opinion of the expert physician, the patient cannot achieve adequate benefit from on-demand treatment of attacks Minority opinion: consider if, despite optimum on-demand treatment, patients experience: • >12 moderate to severe attacks per year • >24 d/y affected by HAE

swellings were absent with androgen therapy but 4 episodes occurred during placebo therapy.[7] A similar beneficial effect is seen with other attenuated androgens, although most evidence is based on danazol therapy.[8] Small open-label studies have shown reduction in attack frequency with both tibolone and oxymetholone.[9,10]

Several open-label, prospective case studies have also shown that a minimum effective dose could be found for most patients to significantly reduce attack frequency.[9–13] One study reported that less than 10% of 141 patients on danazol or stanozolol failed to achieve clinically significant reduction in attacks[14] and, in another retrospective case series of 118 patients, danazol was ineffective in only 5.9%, and reduced attack frequency by 83.8% from 33.3 per year to 5.4 per year.[15] In the patients who did experience breakthrough attacks, reasons included intentional dose reduction, provoking infections or trauma, and interruption of continuous danazol therapy.[15]

Side Effects of Attenuated Androgens

A limitation of attenuated androgens is their side effect profile, varying from liver dysfunction and cardiovascular risk factor modification to menstrual irregularities, virilization, mood alterations, and weight gain.[8] These side effects pose challenges when considering prophylaxis for women, particularly of child-bearing age, as well as children and adolescents. Frequency of adverse effects can be high, with one case series reporting only 21.2% experiencing no adverse effects from danazol.[15] Most evidence relates to danazol, because it has been the most commonly used attenuated androgen.

A Web-based survey of 524 previous or current androgen-using patients with HAE revealed that 59% reported at least moderate weight gain, with other symptoms of anxiety, depression, menstrual abnormalities, virilization, aggression, acne, headaches, and sleep disturbance of at least moderate severity for 1 in 3 patients, although there are limitations with recall bias and a greater proportion of women in both groups.[16]

The effects of weight gain and menstrual irregularities were shown to be dose dependent in a case-control trial; this study also documented a significantly higher prevalence of arterial hypertension (25%) in the androgen-treated group compared with the age-matched control group, which had a higher proportion of men ($P = .02$).[16] The average weight gain reported varies between studies from 2.3 to 4.5 kg[17] up to 10 kg.[18] Reports of up to 45 kg have been documented after 1 year of 800 mg of danazol.[15]

Virilization is a common side effect and has also been shown to be dose dependent.[15,19,20] Transient virilization of female neonates exposed to androgen therapy during pregnancy has been reported,[21] so androgens are not recommended during pregnancy.[4]

Abnormalities in Hepatic Enzymes

Multiple studies show a link between androgen use and increase in hepatic enzyme level, which often reverses on cessation of therapy or dose adjustment[7,11,12,15,21–23]; however, the clinical significance of these changes is not yet established. Of 118 patients on long-term danazol, 14.4% had abnormalities of liver function tests (aspartate transaminase, alanine transaminase, gamma glutamyl transferase [GGT], alkaline phosphatase), and 5 patients subsequently stopped treatment owing to this.[15] Another retrospective study of 46 patients with HAE on long-term danazol showed that 30.4% at year 5 had increases of at least 1 parameter greater than the upper limit of normal, compared with 21.2% of the control HAE group not on androgen therapy;

however, 4 patients had Gilbert disease, and the slight increase in GGT level has been proposed to be linked to increasing age, questioning the clinical significance of these findings.[22] There have also been reports of hepatocyte necrosis with stanozolol.[21]

Liver Neoplasms

There are reports of hepatic neoplasms developing in association with attenuated androgens (mainly danazol); one case series with 46 patients on danazol reported 3 hepatic adenomas and 1 case of multiple benign biliary hamartomas.[15] Another case series of 41 patients on long-term danazol prophylaxis found that 3 out of 11 patients on androgens for more than 10 years developed adenomas.[24] At follow-up, 2 of the 3 adenomas spontaneously resolved between 18 to 26 months after drug cessation.[25] The concern this highlights is that these latter adenomas occurred at doses of danazol commonly used in current practice (albeit at the upper range of recommended dosage), although duration of treatment also appears to be an important risk factor.

There have been 8 reports of hepatocellular carcinoma (HCC) in patients on long-term danazol,[26–33] and 4 in the context of HAE.[26,27,29,30] In 5 cases with details available, histology showed a noncirrhotic background, and alpha fetoprotein level was normal.[26–30] Therefore, ultrasonography is the preferred screening method, although in one report ultrasonography only 9 months before diagnosis was normal.[27] There has also been a case report of hepatocellular focal nodular hyperplasia in a 32-year-old woman on 400 mg/d of danazol for 16 years.[34]

Other ultrasonography abnormalities are less clearly linked to danazol therapy because they are common findings in the general population; in one retrospective study, ultrasonographic findings included cholelithiasis, hepatomegaly, changes in parenchymal reflectivity, liver cysts, and hemangiomas, with no significant difference between patients on and off androgens.[22]

Most studies have shown that there may be dose-dependent increases in hepatic enzyme levels. Current guidelines recommend monitoring these on a 6-monthly basis, alongside alpha fetoprotein and at least annual ultrasonography to assess for the development of hepatic tumors.[4]

Cardiovascular Risks and Lipid Profiles

Androgens have been shown to alter lipid profiles, with an increase in low-density lipoprotein cholesterol (LDL-C) and reduction in high-density lipoprotein cholesterol (HDL-C).[35,36] Most studies of lipid profiles assess danazol, with only 1 cross-sectional study of stanozolol, showing a reduction in HDL-C but no changes in LDL-C.[20]

A study of 37 patients with HAE on long-term danazol compared with 2 control groups (27 HAE controls off danazol and 66 age-matched and sex-matched healthy volunteers) showed that patients with HAE on danazol had significantly higher levels of LDL-C and apolipoprotein B-100, and significantly reduced levels of HDL-C and apolipoprotein A-1 (ApoA-1) compared with both control groups. There was no significant difference in total cholesterol and triglycerides, although patients on danazol had significantly greater disease severity.[36] A follow-up cross-sectional study showed no significant difference in carotid intima thickness between 25 HAE-positive controls and 20 healthy volunteers, despite the HAE group having higher baseline body mass index, creatinine level, and LDL level, and reduced HDL level compared with both control groups.[37]

A placebo-controlled crossover trial assessing danazol safety in 15 healthy white male volunteers showed a 23% reduction in HDL-C level, and 21% reduction in ApoA-1 after 4 weeks of 200 mg/d danazol, with no effect on LDL-C level; these effects subsequently normalized in the placebo arm of the crossover trial[35] (reversibility has also been documented in other trials in patients without HAE[38]). However, the short duration of danazol administration did not reflect the findings in patients with HAE, and it may be that the effects on LDL-C level occur after longer treatment.

What is currently unclear is whether this translates to increased cardiovascular or cerebrovascular risk. There are a few isolated reports of unexpected cardiovascular events during case series,[15] but numbers are too small to identify any statistical significance.[8] However, this issue does require further investigation.

The effect of attenuated androgens on coagulation parameters is not clear at present; a small crossover trial in 15 healthy volunteers showed no change in fibrinolytic or coagulation profiles after 4 weeks of 200 mg/d danazol compared with placebo.[35] Bork and colleagues[15] reported 1 patient with a deep vein thrombosis (DVT) and pulmonary embolism (PE) after 11 months of danazol 200 mg/day, but further details on other risk factors are not elucidated.

Hemorrhagic Cystitis

A potentially underexamined effect of danazol is urinary tract abnormalities; 13 out of 69 patients in a 9-year follow-up on long-term danazol developed hematuria, 10 with hemorrhagic cystitis, seen macroscopically as nonspecific erythema with neovascularity and submucosal telangiectasia. Clinical presentation varied from microscopic hematuria (9 out of 69), macroscopic hematuria (1 out of 69) and irritative bladder symptoms (2 out of 69). In all but 1 patient the changes were reversible on cessation of danazol therapy.[39]

Current Guidelines for the Use of Androgen Therapy as Prophylaxis

Although there are few randomized, double-blinded, placebo-controlled trials, there remains significant evidence that, in a large proportion of patients, attenuated androgen therapy is likely to have a beneficial effect. However, this must be counterbalanced with its significant side effect profile. There has been a gradual reduction in use of androgens as prophylaxis, and doses are not recommended to exceed 2 mg/d for stanozolol, and 200 mg/d for danazol.[2,40] Current guidelines recommend 6-monthly clinical review with complete peripheral blood count, liver enzyme levels, lipid profile, alpha fetoprotein level, and annual abdominal ultrasonography in order to monitor these risks.[4]

C1-INHIBITOR

Plasma-derived C1-inhibitor (C1-INH) concentrates are increasingly used as prophylaxis for patients with HAE. At present, only 1 formulation, Cinryze, is licensed for prophylaxis, and although administration is IV it has rapidly become a significant option in long-term prophylaxis. Recent data has also demonstrated the efficacy of subcutaneous C1-INH, which is likely to be an important future management strategy.[41]

Efficacy

Randomized controlled trials for C1-INH are sparse and include small numbers of patients. A double-blinded, randomized controlled trial showed a positive effect of C1-INH prophylaxis in 6 patients (4 still on androgen therapy). Over 17 days they were given either 5 doses of IV placebo or C1-INH (25 plasma units per kilogram) and crossed over after a minimum 3-week washout period. During C1-INH administration there was greater than a 60% reduction in mean daily scores for peripheral, genital, laryngeal, and abdominal attacks.[42] Another randomized, double-blinded, placebo-controlled crossover trial allocated 22 patients with HAE to either 12 weeks of IV C1-INH 1000 units twice weekly or placebo (normal saline). Other prophylactic agents were continued through the trial. IV C1-INH reduced attack frequency over the 12-week period from 12.73 to 6.36 (*P*<.001), significantly reducing severity and duration of breakthrough attacks.[43]

Subsequent case series[44,45] and larger open-label trials have supported these earlier findings[46]; one large, multicenter, open-label trial of 146 patients receiving 1000 units of C1-INH every 3 to 7 days showed a reduction in attack frequency to 0.19 attacks per month from a historical attack frequency (retrospectively collected) of 3 per month (a 93.7% reduction; *P*<.001). This study also showed a direct correlation between dosing intervals and attack frequency, and that twice weekly dosing had a more favorable response rate compared with weekly dosing.[46] There has also been a study showing that weekly 50 units/kg recombinant C1-INH reduced attack frequency from 0.9 to 0.4 attacks per week (95% confidence interval [CI], 0.28–0.56),[47] which is surprising owing to its shorter circulating half-life than plasma-derived C1-INH.

C1-INH as prophylaxis has been investigated in pediatrics owing to contraindications with androgen therapy. In one crossover, randomized, placebo-controlled trial with 4 children aged 9 to 17 years receiving 1000 units IV C1-INH every 3 to 4 days for 12 weeks, there was a reduction in mean number of attacks from 13 to 7. Subsequently 23 children went on to open-label prophylaxis, which reduced the median monthly attack rate from 3 to 0.39.[48]

A retrospective analysis of clinical trial and compassionate use data during pregnancy showed no drug-related adverse fetal events in the acute and prophylactic use of C1-INH,[49] which seems to be safe and efficacious.[50,51] C1-INH is currently the treatment of choice if long-term prophylactic treatment is needed during pregnancy or breastfeeding.[52]

Dosing and Delivery Route

Cinryze is currently licensed for long-term prophylaxis for HAE at a dose of 1000 units intravenously every 3 or 4 days, with observational evidence supporting the safety and efficacy of home IV infusions by patients[53]; however, prophylaxis may also be delivered by caregivers and medical or nursing agencies.

Ongoing Developments

One study has shown that escalating doses up to 2500 units every 3 to 4 days was effective and well tolerated in patients who were poorly controlled on 1000 units twice weekly.[44] There is also a recently published Phase III double-blind randomized control crossover trial of subcutaneous C1 inhibitor showing higher efficacy compared with historical IV regimens in reducing the number of attacks per month. At the time of writing, the approved dose has yet to be agreed. However, early indications are that trough C1-INH function level correlates strongly with likelihood of angioedema attack. Therefore individual trough-based dose adjustment may enable freedom from attacks for the majority.[41]

Side Effects

Compared with attenuated androgens, C1-INH is well tolerated, as documented by clinical trials assessing its efficacy and safety; in a trial of 22 patients, 3 adverse events were documented that were possibly drug related: fever, pruritus and rash, and lightheadedness.[43] In a pediatric study, 3 adverse events of mild severity were reported: fever, headache and nausea, and infusion site erythema.[48] Large-scale registry and observational data support its high tolerability, with the Berinert Registry reporting a rate of 0.09 events per infusion.[54]

Thromboembolic Events

There have been multiple case reports of thromboembolic events during studies of C1-INH. In an open-label trial of 146 patients, 5 subjects (all with underlying risk factors) experienced thromboembolic events (myocardial infarction, Deep Vein Thrombosis (DVT), 2 cardiovascular accidents, and a pulmonary embolism (PE)); however, none were considered drug related.[46] Although observational data has not clearly documented an increased risk in thrombosis,[54] a physician survey of patients on C1-INH and adverse events noted that 18% (3 out of 17) of patients with a central catheter experienced a thromboembolic event compared with 0.6% of patients without a central catheter.[49] Recent data published from the Berinert Registry reported 2 thrombotic events in 296 subjects and 9148 infusions between 2010 and 2014: 1 myocardial infarction with multiple risk factors thought to be unrelated to C1-INH, and a subclavian DVT in association with an indwelling catheter, giving a total thrombotic event rate of 0.0002 events per infusion.[55] Caution is therefore needed in patients with preexisting prothrombotic risk factors.

Theoretic Viral/Prion Risk

Being derived from human plasma, there is the theoretical risk of blood-borne virus transmission, along with prions; however, to date there is no documented viral transmission risk, or development of neutralizing antibodies.[56]

TRANEXAMIC ACID

Tranexamic acid (TXA) has been used as a prophylactic agent in the past; its efficacy is lower than that of attenuated androgens[5] but its more favorable side effect profile has created a role for its management, predominantly in pediatrics.[40]

There are very few trials of TXA efficacy; early trials seemed to show a moderate effect that has not been corroborated on larger-scale data.[57,58] Sheffer and colleagues[57] conducted a short, randomized, double-blind, placebo-controlled crossover trial in 18 patients receiving either 1 g of TXA or placebo 3 times per day. Six patients failed to enter the crossover period, but, for those who did, TXA significantly reduced attack frequency (20 attacks over 88 months for TXA and 57 attacks over 53 months with placebo; $P<.005$). In a retrospective case series of more than 400 Italian patients, with a subgroup on prophylactic antifibrinolytics (number not specified), TXA only caused significant attack reduction in 25%, with no effect on a further 45%, and more significant improvements being seen with androgen therapy.[14]

Safety Profile and Side Effects

The tolerability and side effect profile of TXA is much better compared with attenuated androgens; common side effects reported include gastrointestinal upset (diarrhea, nausea, and vomiting).[59] There is a theoretic risk of thrombosis, and case reports exist of patients experiencing thrombotic events while on TXA, albeit in association with other risk factors.[60] However, there are no reported increased risks of thromboembolic events, including myocardial infarction and stroke, in large trials and meta-analyses in multiple different clinical contexts (cardiovascular surgery, trauma, obstetrics).[61] Caution is advised in patients who have other risk factors for thrombosis.

Current consensus guidelines do not recommend TXA as first-line prophylaxis, owing to inferior efficacy compared with androgens.[4,62] However, because androgens are contraindicated in the pediatric population, guidelines state that TXA should be considered as first-line prophylaxis, at 20 to 50 mg/kg in 2 to 3 divided doses 'UP TO A MAXIMUM OF 3-6g/DAY', provided there is no personal or family history of thromboembolism.[63] Current guidelines for HAE in women highlight that TXA has been shown to cross the placenta, but there are data reporting no adverse events with its use in the second and third trimesters, although treatment was for shorter duration than is typically seen in the HAE population. Cases therefore need to be considered on an individual basis with discussion of risks and benefits.[52] TXA has been shown to be present in breast milk and therefore should be stopped during breastfeeding.[64]

PROGESTAGENS

Hormonal influences on disease expression of HAE are well established, with one study reporting a worsening of attack frequency at puberty in 62% of 150 women surveyed.[65] Menstruation triggered attacks in 35%, and ovulation in 14%.[65] Estrogens and combined oral contraceptives typically worsen disease for women and should be avoided.[65]

Although there are no randomized controlled trials assessing progestagens as prophylaxis, there are observational data supporting its favorable profile as a contraceptive agent in HAE. One retrospective study in a French cohort of 55 female patients with HAE types 1 to 3 and idiopathic angioedema showed a benefit of oral progestins. Of those on progestin-only pills (POPs), 61.3% had an improvement in symptoms compared with 89.5% of those on the antigonadotrophic progestagens lynestrenol, nomegestrol acetate, and chlormadinone acetate ($P = .013$).[66] However, there was a paradoxic worsening of symptoms in 7 patients in the POP group (on desogestrel, levonorgestrel, and L-norgestrel intrauterine device), which may be from induction of luteal cysts with estrogen production.[67] A retrospective study reported similar rates of success with POPs, with 64% of patients experiencing symptomatic improvement.[65]

Side Effect Profile

Progestagens are typically better tolerated compared with attenuated androgens; however, some androgenic adverse effects can be noted. In Saule and colleagues'[66] study, 30.9% of patients reported mild adverse events, mainly weight gain, symptoms of estrogen deficiency, breakthrough vaginal bleeding, and hyperandrogenism, although these largely resolved on switching to an alternative progestagen.

Use as Prophylaxis

There is a role for progestagens as long-term prophylaxis, either as POPs or as high-dose progestins (eg, 10 mg of norethisterone), but their efficacy is likely inferior to androgens and C1-INH. Owing to some androgenic side effects, they are not recommended in conjunction with attenuated androgens to avoid theoretic amplification of adverse effects. Similarly, they should not be combined with TXA owing to theoretic thrombotic risk,[52] although a recent systematic review reports no increased risk of thrombosis in oral progesterone–only contraceptives, with some limited evidence for possible increased venous thromboembolism risk with injectable progesterones.[68]

SHORT-TERM PROPHYLAXIS
Introduction

Aside from a robust acute attack management plan and long-term prophylaxis if indicated, short-term prophylaxis (STP) is an important aspect of prevention and treatment in patients with HAE. It should be considered during any exposure known to increase attack risk. Such exposures include medical, dental, and surgical procedures; patient-specific events that may trigger swelling, such as stress related to examinations; or events in which swelling may incur extra risk, such as adventure holidays.

Dental procedures and upper airway manipulation have been the focus of attention, owing to the potentially life-threatening consequences of local edema and airway obstruction. One retrospective analysis of 171 patients undergoing tooth extractions reported an incidence of HAE attacks (facial or laryngeal edema) of 21.5% in patients without prophylaxis,[69] typically occurring between 1 and 72 hours after the event (mean, 14.3 hours).[69] One study of different surgical procedures in a German cohort showed risk ranging between 5.7% and 30.5% (CI, 3.5%–35.7%)[70] so STP should be at least considered in all patients undergoing any procedure.

Options for Short-term Prophylaxis

There are no prospective trial data directly comparing different methods of prophylaxis, making STP choices difficult for clinicians. One retrospective survey of C1-INH, Attenuated androgens (AAs), and TXA reported a statistically significant improvement in number of breakthrough attacks with C1-INH as STP (9%), increasing to 36% with danazol and 50% with TXA.[71]

C1 Inhibitor

At present, Cinryze is licensed at a dose of 1000 units within 24 hours of the procedure, and Berinert (another plasma-derived C1-INH) at 1000 units within 6 hours. Retrospective data available on C1-INH as prophylaxis show efficacy, with one trial showing HAE attacks in only 2% (2 out of 91) of various procedures, in which 1000 units were given within the 24 hours before intervention in 96% of the cases (4% were administered different doses).[72] In the study by Bork and colleagues[69] of tooth extractions, 16% of patients experienced an attack after prophylaxis of 500 units C1-INH, and 7.5% of patients after 1000 units ($P<.035$). Recent data published from the Berinert Registry on STP reported a low rate of attacks per infusion of 0.04, 0.06, and 0.11 within 1, 2, and 3 days of the procedure respectively, with median doses of 14.6 IU/kg or 1000 units.[73] However, data were not available on the procedure done, or on baseline attack rate, and no control group was available.[73] Note that, even despite prophylaxis, breakthrough attacks can occur, so availability of on-demand acute treatment is essential.[62]

Attenuated Androgens

There is very little literature on the efficacy of attenuated androgens as STP; one study of 12 patients reported no attacks on 600 mg danazol per day for 4 days before and after maxillodental procedures[74]; however, there were no controls and the numbers are likely to be too small to detect any statistical significance. Current recommended dose of danazol is 2.5 to 10 mg/kg (maximum, 600 mg/d) to be taken daily from 5 days before the procedure and continued until 2 to 3 days postprocedure.[1] If already on androgens, patients may increase the dose 50% to 100% (up to maximum 600 mg/d) over a similar time frame.[4]

Tranexamic Acid

TXA is less used as STP; early small studies showing some efficacy during various dental and nondental procedures[75] have not been reproduced or corroborated. In a retrospective survey of 134 interventions, TXA was the least used STP agent and 3 of the 6 patients on TXA (20–40 mg/kg in 3 divided doses up to a maximum of 3 g) went on to have episodes of edema.[71] Although documented efficacy is limited, TXA is still recommended as an option should no other choice be readily available.[1]

There has also been documented use of a bradykinin B2 receptor antagonist as STP for dental extraction with success; however, given its short half-life, the biological rationale is unclear, and it is not currently recommended in guidelines.[76]

SUMMARY

There are a variety of evidence-based options for both long-term prophylaxis and STP, with only indirect comparisons of agents in studies to date.[77] Each agent has its benefits and drawbacks in the contexts of efficacy, tolerability, inconvenience, and cost, and better, and more numerous, options for children and pregnant women are particularly needed. There are several new agents undergoing further clinical trials at present that are promising in potentially overcoming some of the limitations with agents currently in everyday use.

REFERENCES

1. Betschel S, Badiou J, Binkley K, et al. Canadian hereditary angioedema guideline. Allergy Asthma Clin Immunol 2014;10(1):50.
2. Craig T, Aygören-Pürsün E, Bork K, et al. WAO guideline for the management of hereditary angioedema. World Allergy Organ J 2012;5:182–99.
3. Zuraw BL, Banerji A, Bernstein JA, et al. US Hereditary Angioedema Association Medical Advisory Board 2013 recommendations for the management of hereditary angioedema due to C1 inhibitor deficiency. US Hereditary Angioedema Association Medical Advisory Board. J Allergy Clin Immunol Pract 2013;1(5): 458–67.
4. Cicardi M, Bork K, Caballero T, et al. Evidence-based recommendations for the therapeutic management of angioedema owing to hereditary C1 inhibitor deficiency: consensus report of an international working group. Allergy 2012;67: 147–57.
5. Zuraw BL, Davis DK, Castaldo AJ, et al. Tolerability and effectiveness of 17-α-alkylated androgen therapy for hereditary angioedema: a re-examination. J Allergy Clin Immunol Pract 2016;4:948–55.e15.
6. Gelfand JA, Sherins RJ, Alling DW, et al. Treatment of hereditary angioedema with danazol. Reversal of clinical and biochemical abnormalities. N Engl J Med 1976; 295:1444–8.
7. Sheffer AL, Fearon DT, Austen KF. Methyltestosterone therapy in hereditary angioedema. Ann Intern Med 1977;86:306–8.
8. Riedl MA. Critical appraisal of androgen use in hereditary angioedema: a systematic review. Ann Allergy Asthma Immunol 2015;114:281–8.e287.
9. Ott HW, Mattle V, Hadziomerovic D, et al. Treatment of hereditary angioneurotic oedema (HANE) with tibolone. Clin Endocrinol (Oxf) 2007;66:180–4.
10. Sheffer AL, Fearon DT, Austen KF. Clinical and biochemical effects of impeded androgen (oxymetholone) therapy of hereditary angioedema. J Allergy Clin Immunol 1979;64:275–80.
11. Rothbach C, Green RL, Levine MI, et al. Prophylaxis of attacks of hereditary angioedema. Am J Med 1979;66:681–3.
12. Santaella ML, Martinó A. Hereditary and acquired angioedema: experience with patients in Puerto Rico. P R Health Sci J 2004;23:13–8.
13. Sheffer AL, Fearon DT, Austen KF. Clinical and biochemical effects of stanozolol therapy for hereditary angioedema. J Allergy Clin Immunol 1981;68:181–7.
14. Cicardi M, Zingale L. How do we treat patients with hereditary angioedema. Transfus Apher Sci 2003;29:221–7.
15. Bork K, Bygum A, Hardt J. Benefits and risks of danazol in hereditary angioedema: a long-term survey of 118 patients. Ann Allergy Asthma Immunol 2008; 100:153–61.

16. Cicardi M, Castelli R, Zingale LC, et al. Side effects of long-term prophylaxis with attenuated androgens in hereditary angioedema: comparison of treated and untreated patients. J Allergy Clin Immunol 1997;99:194–6.

17. Hosea SW, Santaella ML, Brown EJ, et al. Long-term therapy of hereditary angioedema with danazol. Ann Intern Med 1980;93:809–12.

18. Zotter Z, Veszeli N, Csuka D, et al. Frequency of the virilising effects of attenuated androgens reported by women with hereditary angioedema. Orphanet J Rare Dis 2014;9:205.

19. Sheffer AL, Fearon DT, Austen KF. Hereditary angioedema: a decade of management with stanozolol. J Allergy Clin Immunol 1987;80:855–60.

20. Sloane DE, Lee CW, Sheffer AL. Hereditary angioedema: safety of long-term stanozolol therapy. J Allergy Clin Immunol 2007;120:654–8.

21. Cicardi M, Bergamaschini L, Cugno M, et al. Long-term treatment of hereditary angioedema with attenuated androgens: a survey of a 13-year experience. J Allergy Clin Immunol 1991;87:768–73.

22. Farkas H, Czaller I, Csuka D, et al. The effect of long-term danazol prophylaxis on liver function in hereditary angioedema-a longitudinal study. Eur J Clin Pharmacol 2010;66:419–26.

23. Cicardi M, Bergamaschini L, Tucci A, et al. Morphologic evaluation of the liver in hereditary angioedema patients on long-term treatment with androgen derivatives. J Allergy Clin Immunol 1983;72:294–8.

24. Bork K, Pitton M, Harten P, et al. Hepatocellular adenomas in patients taking danazol for hereditary angio-oedema. Lancet 1999;353:1066–7.

25. Bork K, Schneiders V. Danazol-induced hepatocellular adenoma in patients with hereditary angio-oedema. J Hepatol 2002;36:707–9.

26. Thoufeeq MH, Ishtiaq J, Abuzakouk M. Danazol-induced hepatocellular carcinoma in a patient with hereditary angioedema. J Gastrointest Cancer 2012; 43(Suppl 1):S280–2.

27. Berkel AE, Bouman DE, Schaafsma MR, et al. Hepatocellular carcinoma after danazol treatment for hereditary angio-oedema. Neth J Med 2014;72:380–2.

28. Confavreux C, Sève P, Broussolle C, et al. Danazol-induced hepatocellular carcinoma. QJM 2003;96:317–8.

29. Crampon D, Barnoud R, Durand M, et al. Danazol therapy: an unusual aetiology of hepatocellular carcinoma. J Hepatol 1998;29:1035–6.

30. Rahal S, Gilabert M, Ries P, et al. Hepatocellular carcinoma in a noncirrhotic liver after long-term use of danazol for hereditary angioedema. Case Rep Oncol 2014; 7:825–7.

31. Middleton C, McCaughan GW, Painter DM, et al. Danazol and hepatic neoplasia: a case report. Aust N Z J Med 1989;19:733–5.

32. Buamah PK. An apparent danazol-induced primary hepatocellular carcinoma: case report. J Surg Oncol 1985;28:114–6.

33. Weill BJ, Menkès CJ, Cormier C, et al. Hepatocellular carcinoma after danazol therapy. J Rheumatol 1988;15:1447–9.

34. Helsing P, Nielsen EW. Hepatocellular focal nodular hyperplasia after danazol treatment for hereditary angio-oedema. Acta Derm Venereol 2006;86:272–3.

35. Birjmohun RS, Kees Hovingh G, Stroes ES, et al. Effects of short-term and long-term danazol treatment on lipoproteins, coagulation, and progression of atherosclerosis: two clinical trials in healthy volunteers and patients with hereditary angioedema. Clin Ther 2008;30:2314–23.

36. Széplaki G, Varga L, Valentin S, et al. Adverse effects of danazol prophylaxis on the lipid profiles of patients with hereditary angioedema. J Allergy Clin Immunol 2005;115:864–9.

37. Szegedi R, Széplaki G, Varga L, et al. Long-term danazol prophylaxis does not lead to increased carotid intima-media thickness in hereditary angioedema patients. Atherosclerosis 2008;198:184–91.

38. Allen JK, Fraser IS. Cholesterol, high density lipoprotein and danazol. J Clin Endocrinol Metab 1981;53:149–52.

39. Andriole GL, Brickman C, Lack EE, et al. Danazol-induced cystitis: an undescribed source of hematuria in patients with hereditary angioneurotic edema. J Urol 1986;135:44–6.

40. Longhurst H, Cicardi M. Hereditary angio-oedema. Lancet 2012;379:474–81.

41. Longhurst H, Cicardi M, Craig T, et al. Prevention of Hereditary Angioedema Attacks with a Subcutaneous C1 inhibitor. N Engl J Med 2017;376(12):1131–40.

42. Waytes AT, Rosen FS, Frank MM. Treatment of hereditary angioedema with a vapor-heated C1 inhibitor concentrate. N Engl J Med 1996;334:1630–4.

43. Zuraw BL, Busse PJ, White M, et al. Nanofiltered C1 inhibitor concentrate for treatment of hereditary angioedema. N Engl J Med 2010;363:513–22.

44. Bernstein JA, Manning ME, Li H, et al. Escalating doses of C1 esterase inhibitor (CINRYZE) for prophylaxis in patients with hereditary angioedema. J Allergy Clin Immunol Pract 2014;2:77–84.

45. Bork K, Hardt J. Hereditary angioedema: long-term treatment with one or more injections of C1 inhibitor concentrate per week. Int Arch Allergy Immunol 2011; 154:81–8.

46. Zuraw BL, Kalfus I. Safety and efficacy of prophylactic nanofiltered C1-inhibitor in hereditary angioedema. Am J Med 2012;125:938.e1-7.

47. Reshef A, Moldovan D, Obtulowicz K, et al. Recombinant human C1 inhibitor for the prophylaxis of hereditary angioedema attacks: a pilot study. Allergy 2013;68: 118–24.

48. Lumry W, Manning ME, Hurewitz DS, et al. Nanofiltered C1-esterase inhibitor for the acute management and prevention of hereditary angioedema attacks due to C1-inhibitor deficiency in children. J Pediatr 2013;162:1017–22.e1-2.

49. Kalaria S, Craig T. Assessment of hereditary angioedema treatment risks. Allergy Asthma Proc 2013;34:519–22.

50. Baker JW, Craig TJ, Riedl MA, et al. Nanofiltered C1 esterase inhibitor (human) for hereditary angioedema attacks in pregnant women. Allergy Asthma Proc 2013; 34:162–9.

51. Gorman PJ. Hereditary angioedema and pregnancy: a successful outcome using C1 esterase inhibitor concentrate. Can Fam Physician 2008;54:365–6.

52. Caballero T, Farkas H, Bouillet L, et al. International consensus and practical guidelines on the gynecologic and obstetric management of female patients with hereditary angioedema caused by C1 inhibitor deficiency. J Allergy Clin Immunol 2012;129:308–20.

53. Levi M, Choi G, Picavet C, et al. Self-administration of C1-inhibitor concentrate in patients with hereditary or acquired angioedema caused by C1-inhibitor deficiency. J Allergy Clin Immunol 2006;117:904–8.

54. Busse P, Bygum A, Edelman J, et al. Safety of C1-esterase inhibitor in acute and prophylactic therapy of hereditary angioedema: findings from the ongoing international Berinert patient registry. J Allergy Clin Immunol Pract 2015;3:213–9.

55. Riedl MA, Bygum A, Lumry W, et al. Safety and usage of C1-inhibitor in hereditary angioedema: Berinert Registry data. J Allergy Clin Immunol Pract 2016;4(5):963.

56. Bork K, Steffensen I, Machnig T. Treatment with C1-esterase inhibitor concentrate in type I or II hereditary angioedema: a systematic literature review. Allergy Asthma Proc 2013;34:312–27.

57. Sheffer AL, Austen KF, Rosen FS. Tranexamic acid therapy in hereditary angioneurotic edema. N Engl J Med 1972;287:452–4.

58. Frank MM, Sergent JS, Kane MA, et al. Epsilon aminocaproic acid therapy of hereditary angioneurotic edema. A double-blind study. N Engl J Med 1972;286:808–12.

59. Joint Formulary Committee. British National Formulary.72. London: BMJ Group and Pharmaceutical Press; 2015.

60. Günaldi M, Helvaci A, Yildirim ND, et al. Acute myocardial infarction in a patient with hemophilia A and factor V Leiden mutation. Cardiol J 2009;16:458–61.

61. Ng W, Jerath A, Wąsowicz M. Tranexamic acid: a clinical review. Anaesthesiol Intensive Ther 2015;47:339–50.

62. Bowen T, Cicardi M, Farkas H, et al. 2010 International consensus algorithm for the diagnosis, therapy and management of hereditary angioedema. Allergy Asthma Clin Immunol 2010;6:24.

63. Farkas H, Martinez-Saguer I, Bork K, et al. International consensus on the diagnosis and management of pediatric patients with hereditary angioedema with C1 inhibitor deficiency. Allergy 2017;72(2):300–13.

64. Bouillet L. Hereditary angioedema in women. Allergy Asthma Clin Immunol 2010;6:17.

65. Bouillet L, Longhurst H, Boccon-Gibod I, et al. Disease expression in women with hereditary angioedema. Am J Obstet Gynecol 2008;199:484.e1-4.

66. Saule C, Boccon-Gibod I, Fain O, et al. Benefits of progestin contraception in non-allergic angioedema. Clin Exp Allergy 2013;43:475–82.

67. Longhurst HJ. Hereditary and other orphan angioedemas: a new prophylactic option at last? Clin Exp Allergy 2013;43:380–2.

68. Tepper NK, Whiteman MK, Marchbanks PA, et al. Progestin-only contraception and thromboembolism: a systematic review. Contraception 2016;94:678–700.

69. Bork K, Hardt J, Staubach-Renz P, et al. Risk of laryngeal edema and facial swellings after tooth extraction in patients with hereditary angioedema with and without prophylaxis with C1 inhibitor concentrate: a retrospective study. Oral Surg Oral Med Oral Pathol Oral Radiol Endod 2011;112:58–64.

70. Aygoren-Pursun E, Martinez Saguer I, Kreuz W, et al. Risk of angioedema following invasive or surgical procedures in HAE type I and II–the natural history. Allergy 2013;68:1034–9.

71. Farkas H, Zotter Z, Csuka D, et al. Short-term prophylaxis in hereditary angioedema due to deficiency of the C1-inhibitor–a long-term survey. Allergy 2012;67:1586–93.

72. Grant JA, White MV, Li HH, et al. Preprocedural administration of nanofiltered C1 esterase inhibitor to prevent hereditary angioedema attacks. Allergy Asthma Proc 2012;33:348–53.

73. Magerl M, Frank M, Lumry W, et al. Short-term prophylactic use of C1-inhibitor concentrate in hereditary angioedema: findings from an international patient registry. Ann Allergy Asthma Immunol 2017;118(1):110–2.

74. Farkas H, Gyeney L, Gidofalvy E, et al. The efficacy of short-term danazol prophylaxis in hereditary angioedema patients undergoing maxillofacial and dental procedures. J Oral Maxillofac Surg 1999;57:404–8.

75. Sheffer AL, Fearon DT, Austen KF, et al. Tranexamic acid: preoperative prophy-lactic therapy for patients with hereditary angioneurotic edema. J Allergy Clin Im-munol 1977;60:38–40.
76. Angeletti C, Angeletti PM, Mastrobuono F, et al. Bradykinin B2 receptor antago-nist off label use in short-term prophylaxis in hereditary angioedema. Int J Immu-nopathol Pharmacol 2014;27:653–9.
77. Costantino G, Casazza G, Bossi I, et al. Long-term prophylaxis in hereditary angio-edema: a systematic review. BMJ Open 2012;2(4) [pii: e000524].

Hereditary Angioedema with Normal C1 Inhibitor
Update on Evaluation and Treatment

Markus Magerl, MD[a],*, Anastasios E. Germenis, MD, PhD[b],
Coen Maas, PhD[c], Marcus Maurer, MD[a]

KEYWORDS

• Hereditary angioedema • Factor XII • Plasmin • Mutation • Bradykinin • C1-inhibitor

KEY POINTS

- Clinically, hereditary angioedema with normal C1 inhibitor (HAE-nC1) is similar to hereditary angioedema caused by C1 inhibitor (C1-INH) deficiency, but not identical. About a quarter of HAE-nC1 cases are attributed to mutations in the F12 gene; in three-quarters of the cases the pathomechanism is still widely unknown.
- Swelling attacks in patients with HAE-nC1 are thought to be caused by bradykinin.
- As of now, there are no routine laboratory tests to confirm the diagnosis of HAE-nC1, so the diagnosis is based on history and clinical criteria.

INTRODUCTION

Hereditary angioedema (HAE) was first described by Dinkelacker[1] and Quincke[2] in 1882 and a few years later by Osler[3] as recurrent angioedema with a positive family history. In 1963, Donaldson[4] identified the "absence of serum inhibitor of C′ 1-esterase" (C1-INH) as the underlying disorder of type 1 HAE caused by C1-INH deficiency (HAE-C1-INH). Not long after, Rosen and colleagues[5] described a second genetic variant of HAE-C1-INH, which is caused by deficient functional activity of

Conflicts of interest: M. Magerl has received consultancy/honorarium fees from Shire, Viropharma, CSL Behring, and Sobi. A.E. Germenis has received research support from Shire (grant no: IIR-GRC-000905), Amgen, and Novartis; has received consultancy fees from Shire; has received lecture fees from Novartis and Amgen; and has received travel support from Shire. C. Maas is consultant to Shire, Pharming. M. Maurer has received research support, consultancy/lecture fees, and/or travel support from Biocryst, CSL Behring, and Shire/Dyax/Viropharma.
[a] Department of Dermatology and Allergy, Allergie-Centrum-Charité/ECARF, Charité - Universitätsmedizin Berlin, Charitéplatz 1, Berlin 10117, Germany; [b] Department of Immunology and Histocompatibility, Faculty of Medicine, School of Health Sciences, University of Thessaly, Panepistimiou 3, GR-41500 Biopolis, Larissa, Greece; [c] Department of Clinical Chemistry and Haematology, University Medical Center Utrecht, Heidelberglaan 100, Utrecht 3584CX, The Netherlands
* Corresponding author.
E-mail address: markus.magerl@charite.de

Immunol Allergy Clin N Am 37 (2017) 571–584
http://dx.doi.org/10.1016/j.iac.2017.04.004
0889-8561/17/© 2017 Elsevier Inc. All rights reserved.

immunology.theclinics.com

C1-INH. Bradykinin, which results from activation of the contact system, was first suspected in the 1960s to be the mediator responsible for the signs and symptoms of both types of HAE-C1-INH,[6,7] and this was proved in the 1990s.[8] In 2000, a new form of HAE with normal C1-INH was first described, independently from each other, by Binkley and colleagues[9] and Bork and colleagues.[10] Initially, this new type of HAE was called HAE type 3. Its current designation is HAE with normal C1-INH (HAE-nC1). Four mutations in the FXII gene have been described to be linked to HAEnC1,[11–13] all of which affect the proline-rich region (PRR) of the FXII protein. HAE-nC1 in patients with a mutation in the FXII gene is designated as HAE with F12 gene mutation (HAE-FXII). However, in most patients with HAE-nC1, no mutation in the FXII gene can be found, and the pathogenesis remains unclear (HAE unknown [HAE-UNK]).

THE PATHOPHYSIOLOGY OF HEREDITARY ANGIOEDEMA WITH NORMAL C1 INHIBITOR

Swelling attacks in patients with HAE-C1-INH are brought about by activation of the contact system and the subsequent generation of bradykinin, which causes extravasation by activating the bradykinin 2 receptor. This pathomechanism is thought to also be involved in HAE-nC1. The contact system, a side-branch enzyme system of the coagulation system, consists of factor XII (FXII), plasma prekallikrein (PPK), and high-molecular-weight kininogen (HK). These factors generate spontaneous enzymatic activity when they assemble on surface materials (**Fig. 1**). The contact system is linked to the coagulation system by factor XI (FXI): both PPK and FXI are complexed with HK in the systemic circulation. Surfaces that activate the contact system can be non-natural, such as the inner surfaces of extracorporeal membrane oxygenation devices,[14] or the mineral particulate kaolin, which is commonly used in coagulation diagnostics.[15] However, several endogenously occurring triggering materials for contact system activation have been identified. These materials include extracellular nucleic acids,[16] platelet polyphosphate,[17] mast cell–derived heparin,[18] and aggregated proteins,[19] including toxic aggregates that are formed by amyloid-β peptide.[20] During contact activation, FXII lands on the activating surface and becomes spontaneously active. Both PPK and FXI are presented for activation by activated FXII (FXIIa). Several reciprocal cleavage steps between FXIIa and plasma kallikrein (PK) are needed to generate a burst of enzyme activity. HK is needed to concentrate these factors on

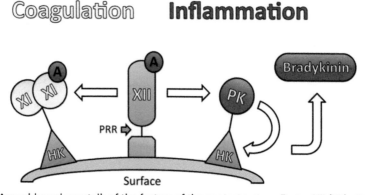

Fig. 1. Assembly and crosstalk of the factors of the contact system. Factor XII (XII) attaches to the surface and becomes active (FXIIa). Next, it can activate PPK to active plasma kallikrein (PK). Simultaneously, FXIIa activates factor XI (FXIa). HK mediates assembly of PK and FXI on the contact surface. Ultimately, bradykinin is liberated by PK from HK.

the activating surface (see **Fig. 1**). During this reaction, active PK can cleave its own cofactor HK to release bradykinin. C1-INH is the major inhibitor of FXIIa, PK, and FXIa, which explains why excessive bradykinin production is seen in C1-INH deficiency. It is generally assumed that coagulation and bradykinin production always take place simultaneously. However, bradykinin can be produced in the absence of clotting.[19] This process depends on the specific physical properties of the activator of the contact system. In general, insoluble particles trigger both coagulation and bradykinin production, whereas anionic polymers only trigger bradykinin production.[21] The underlying trigger for contact system activation in HAE remains elusive, but there is a striking lack of thrombotic features during the bradykinin-driven attacks of HAE-C1-INH,[22] which suggests that the trigger for contact activation does not strongly trigger coagulation.

As of now, there is no direct evidence that swelling attacks in patients with HAE-nC1, but without F12 mutations, are generally caused by contact system activation and bradykinin. However, there are several indirect lines of evidence in support of this: for example, plasma bradykinin levels were reported to be increased in patients with idiopathic nonhistaminergic angioedema.[23] Also, kininogen consumption (which is considered to reflect bradykinin production) has been repeatedly observed in patients with anaphylaxis[24] and is particularly pronounced in patients with anaphylaxis who develop angioedema during their attacks.[25] These findings are seemingly contradictory to studies in which plasma bradykinin levels in patients with histaminergic angioedema are within normal range.[26] A likely explanation for this is that the circulating half-life of bradykinin is very short, whereas cleavage products of kininogen are expected to circulate much longer.

Recent studies suggest that plasmin is involved in the pathogenesis of HAE-nC1. Plasmin is the main enzyme of the fibrinolytic system and is responsible for the degradation of fibrin polymers in blood clots. To achieve this goal, plasmin is locally generated on the fibrin strands. Intriguingly, plasmin is also generated on the surface of endothelial cells. This process can occur in the absence of fibrin; for example, during tissue hypoxia.[27] Plasmin importantly interacts with the contact system: (1) plasmin can cleave FXII, which leads to its activation[28]; (2) angioedema is seen as a side-effect of therapies that induce plasmin activity.[29,30] During this treatment, FXII is activated in plasma.[31] Evidence that plasmin is a relevant player in the pathogenesis of HAE-nC1 comes from studies that show that levels of PAI-2, a protein that controls plasmin activity, are decreased during attacks.[32] Also, patients with HAE-nC1 reportedly benefit from treatment with tranexamic acid, a selective and direct inhibitor of plasmin activation and activity.[33] Tranexamic acid strongly inhibited spontaneous plasmin activity in the plasma of patients with HAE-nC1 who benefited from this therapy.[34] Increased plasmin activity has also been described in HAE-C1-INH,[35,36] in which it reportedly correlates with increased consumption of HK and disease activity.[37] Increased plasmin activity and contact system activity are also seen in anaphylaxis, in particular when patients develop angioedema.[25,38]

THE GENETICS OF HEREDITARY ANGIOEDEMA WITH NORMAL C1 INHIBITOR

About a quarter of HAE-nC1 cases are attributed to mutations in the F12 gene located in chromosome 5 (5q33-qter) and encoding for coagulation factor XII (Hageman factor, FXII). Up to now, four F12 mutations have been identified and are thought to be causal for HAE-nC1 based on their cosegregation patterns.[39] All of them are located in the proline-rich linker peptide between the Kringle and trypsinlike serine protease

(Tryp-SPc) domains of the FXII protein[39]; these are two distinct missense mutations on exon 9, resulting in threonine-to-lysine (Thr328Lys) and threonine-to-arginine (Thr328Arg) substitutions,[11] a large deletion of 72 bp (c.971_1018 + 24del72) located at the exon 9/intron 9 border,[12] and a duplication of 18 bp (c.892_909dup) causing the repeated presence of 6 amino acids (p.298–303) in the same region.[13] The Thr328Lys substitution is the most common and has been identified in clinically affected as well as symptom-free individuals from numerous families.[11,12,40,41] The Thr328Arg replacement has been found only in two German families,[11] the large deletion in two unrelated families of Turkish origin,[12] and the c.892_909dup in a Hungarian family.[13] HAE in patients with HAE-nC1 with one of these F12 mutations is designated HAE-nC1 with FXII mutation (HAE-FXII). HAE in patients with HAE-nC1 without one of these F12 mutations is called HAE-UNK.[42] The inheritance pattern is assumed to be auto-somal dominant for both HAE-FXII and HAE-UNK.

Initially, it was suggested that F12 mutations confer a putative gain of FXII function leading to upregulation of contact system activation and increased bradykinin forma-tion.[43] However, subsequent evidence indicated that the Thr328Lys mutation does not cause a gain of function of FXII.[44] Recent studies have focused on the effects of HAE-FXII F12 mutations on the function of the PRR, where all of them are located. Essentially, this flexible amino-acid sequence (which is unique to FXII) connects the surface-binding domains of FXII to its protease domain. The 309 threonine residue is a target for O-linked glycosylation and displays aberrant glycosylation in T309K and T309R.[45] As a result, the PRR is less negatively charged and the overall protein size of the mutant FXII molecule is reduced and develops an enhanced capacity for spontaneous activation on dextran sulfate, a non-natural negatively charged model polymer that can activate the contact system. Also, the HAE-FXII mutants T309K, T309K, and c.971_1018 + 24del72* introduce one or more cleavage sites into the fac-tor XII molecule that are normally not present. Of note, FXII activation during activation on a negatively charged surface or on endothelial cells requires cleavage by PK.[46] Sur-prisingly, the cleavage sites that are newly introduced by HAE-FXII mutations are insensitive to PK,[47] suggesting that another enzyme is involved in the bradykinin-forming mechanism during angioedema attacks in HAE-FXII. Further studies on the HAE-FXII mutations T309K, T309K, and c.971_1018 + 24del72* revealed that all newly introduced cleavage sites strongly amplify the rate of mutant FXII activation by plasmin, rendering C1-INH ineffective at preventing excessive bradykinin produc-tion.[47] Lysine analogues (tranexamic acid) interfere with this pathologic mechanism, which may explain, at least in part, their mechanism of action in the treatment of patients with HAE-FXII.

Very recently, two F12 mutations (c1681-1G/A [intron 13] and c1027G/C [exon 10]), previously identified in association with FXII deficiency, were reported in pa-tients with idiopathic nonhistaminergic angioedema, one of which was a de novo mutation[48] and the F12 to 46C/T polymorphism was recognized as a modifier of the clinical phenotype of HAE-C1-INH.[49] This polymorphism is located in the pro-moter region of the F12 gene, four nucleotides before the initiation codon (ATG, methionine), creating a new initiation codon (ATG) for transcription of the messenger RNA and a frameshift that produces a truncated protein. The T allele destroys the Kozak consensus sequence (GCCAGCCATGG) for translation initiation signaling and prevents proper recognition of the translation initiation site,[50,51] which raises the question of whether the presence of all F12 alterations considered so far respon-sible for HAE are isolated or are expressed in tandem either with F12 polymorphisms or with functional alterations of other genes involved in the function and/or the degradation of bradykinin.

The genetic basis of HAE-UNK remains to be determined and may involve isolated or combined deficiencies in the three major enzymes that degrade bradykinin, namely carboxypeptidase N, angiotensin-converting enzyme (ACE), and aminopeptidase P.[52,53]

CLINICAL FEATURES OF HEREDITARY ANGIOEDEMA WITH NORMAL C1 INHIBITOR

Similar to HAE-C1-INH, patients with HAE-nC1 experience angioedema attacks of the skin, gastrointestinal tract, and airways. The episodes are transient and generally separated by intervals of complete remission. Individual HAE-nC1 attacks are indistinguishable from HAE-C1-INH attacks. However, HAE-nC1 is different from HAE-C1-INH in many aspects, and the subgroups of HAE-nC1, HAE-FXII, and HAE-UNK also show differences.

The mean age of onset of HAE-nC1 symptoms is reported to be 26.8 years (range, 1–68 years),[54] which is considerably later than in HAE-C1-INH (mean, 12 years; range, 1–79 years; unpublished data from 458 patients, Magerl, 2016). Patients with HAE-FXII are younger at the onset of disease than patients with HAE-UNK. For HAE-FXII, Bork and colleagues,[55] Deroux and colleagues,[56] and Piñero-Saavedra and colleagues[57] found a mean age of onset of 20.3, 21, and 19.9 years, respectively. In contrast, patients with HAE-UNK reportedly develop their first symptoms at a mean age of 29.6 years (range, 1–80 years).[55]

HAE-nC1 predominantly affects women, with only a limited number of affected male patients described.[54,56–59] This sex imbalance seems to be more pronounced in HAE-FXII, in which 76% to 98.5% of patients are female.[55–57] In HAE-nC1, male patients are more likely to be asymptomatic.[11,56] Comparable with HAE-C1-INH, estrogens are frequent triggers of attacks in HAE-nC1. Some female patients reproducibly develop swellings at times of increased exposure to estrogen and are free of symptoms when they are not pregnant or taking an estrogen-containing medicine.[9] In other patients, the role of estrogen is less pronounced or does not influence disease activity, as is predominantly seen in patients with HAE-UNK. Bork and colleagues[55] reported that a significantly higher rate of women with HAE-FXII than with HAE-UNK experienced exacerbation or initial onset of symptoms on oral contraceptive intake, and a similar observation was made during pregnancy. Similar to HAE-C1-INH, attacks in patients with HAE-FXII can be triggered by mechanical trauma, including dental procedures.[60]

In general, patients with HAE-nC1 have more disease-free intervals, and the average frequency of attacks is lower, compared with patients with HAE-C1-INH.[54,56,57,61,62] Patients with HAE-nC1, compared with patients with HAE-C1-INH, predominantly develop facial swellings, whereas swellings at the extremities are less frequent, and genital swellings are rare.[54] Tongue swellings are much more common in HAE-nC1 than in HAE-C1-INH, primarily in HAE-UNK. Abdominal attacks in HAE-C1-INH are less common compared with HAE-C1-INH, especially in HAE-UNK.[55–57,59,62,63] Rates of laryngeal edema in HAE-nC1 vary between studies.[55,57,62] Deaths by suffocation caused by laryngeal edema and/or tongue swellings have been reported.[54,55] Multilocation attacks in HAE-nC1 have been described as less common compared with HAE-C1-INH.[54,64]

Almost all patients with HAE-C1-INH report the occurrence of prodromes, including unspecific symptoms such as fatigue, malaise, short temper, restlessness, and sadness but also erythema marginatum as a specific sign.[65–67] In contrast, prodromes are rare in HAE-nC1. Fatigue and chest discomfort have been observed in only very few patients.[57] Several investigators have explicitly negated the occurrence of erythema marginatum in patients with HAE-nC1.[41,54,56,68] Urticarial whealing in patients with HAE is not seen more frequently than in the general population, either in HAE-C1-INH or in HAE-nC1[69]; that is, a history of urticaria is possible but a co-occurrence of wheals and HAE symptoms is very unlikely. In HAE-nC1, hemorrhages as sequelae have been observed in some patients one or two days after the onset of the swellings, limited to the sites of the angioedema.[54,57]

DIAGNOSIS AND DIFFERENTIAL DIAGNOSIS OF HEREDITARY ANGIOEDEMA WITH NORMAL C1 INHIBITOR
Diagnosis

The diagnostic work-up of HAE-C1-INH is usually straightforward. The history and pattern of signs and symptoms are typical and prompt the assessment of levels of C4 and C1-INH as well as its function. In rare cases, genetic testing may be needed to confirm the diagnosis. Nevertheless, patients with HAE-C1-INH are commonly misdiagnosed, most frequently with allergic angioedema and appendicitis, resulting in long delays in the correct diagnosis.[70,71]

In contrast, the diagnosis of HAE-nC1 is more challenging. Patients with HAE-nC1 present with a history of recurrent angioedema in the absence of concomitant hives; however, the history and symptom pattern are much more variable than in HAE C1-INH. C1-INH level and function, C1q, and C4 are normal. The diagnosis of HAE-FXII requires the demonstration of a mutation in the F12 gene. The diagnosis of HAE-UNK requires a positive family history; that is, one or more family members also affected with these symptoms. As of now, there are no routine laboratory tests to confirm the diagnosis of HAE-nC1.[61,72] Additional emphasis should be given to the clinical features of HAE-nC1 mentioned earlier, such as female sex, the predilection to be exacerbated by estrogens, and the tendency to involve the face, tongue, and upper airway.[72]

Differential Diagnosis

The differential diagnoses of HAE-nC1 include hereditary and acquired forms of recurrent angioedema caused by C1-INH deficiency, recurrent mast cell mediator–mediated angioedema, and nonhereditary recurrent angioedema of unknown causes. Of note, not all recurrent swellings are angioedema and several medical conditions can present with swellings that resemble angioedema. These conditions include but are not limited to acute contact dermatitis, drug rash with eosinophilia and systemic symptoms, dermatomyositis, morbus morbihan, superior vena cava syndrome, hypothyroidism, subcutaneous emphysema, and orofacial granulomatosis.[73]

HAE-C1-INH is similar to HAE-nC1, in terms of history and clinical course. Careful history taking may help to distinguish HAE-nC1 from HAE-C1-INH: the presence of prodromes (primarily erythema marginatum), frequent abdominal attacks, sparse tongue swellings, and no obvious preponderance of women in the family suggest HAE-C1-INH. HAE-C1-INH is readily excluded by measuring antigenic and functional levels of C1-INH and C4. Recurrent angioedema caused by acquired C1-INH deficiency can be excluded by measuring antigenic and functional levels of C1-INH, as well as C1q and C4. It usually starts after the 40th year of life, and the family history is negative. ACE inhibitor–induced angioedema, similar to HAE-nC1, comes predominantly with recurrent swellings of the tongue, lips, and face, but patients do not report prodromes or that other family members are affected.[74] As reported for HAE-C1-INH, ACE inhibitors can also trigger attacks in HAE-nC1 and may in rare cases reveal a so-far silent HAE.[57,60,68,75] A similar trigger function in HAE-nC1 was also reported for the intake of angiotensin II type 1 receptor blockers.[60,76]

Recurrent mast cell mediator–mediated angioedema is a frequent sign in most types of chronic urticaria.[72] Some patients with chronic spontaneous urticaria show exclusively angioedema (and never have hives). To exclude recurrent angioedema caused by chronic spontaneous urticaria, a trial of continuous high-dose (up to 4-fold standard dose) second-generation H1 antihistamine therapy for least 1 month and an interval expected to be associated with three or more attacks of angioedema is helpful.[72] Approximately 30% to 60% of patients with urticaria can be expected to achieve complete symptom control with this approach.[77,78] Failure to show improvement does not prove that chronic spontaneous urticaria is not the underlying cause. Another theranostic approach is the use of omalizumab (anti–immunoglobulin E), which benefit most patients with recurrent angioedema caused by chronic spontaneous urticaria, with and without hives.[79–85]

TREATMENT OF HEREDITARY ANGIOEDEMA WITH NORMAL C1 INHIBITOR

No prospective, randomized controlled studies have been performed so far in patients with HAE-nC1, and there are, therefore, no licensed treatments available as of now. However, several observational studies have assessed various medications for the treatment of HAE-nC1, although most of these studies do not clearly distinguish between HAE-UNK and HAE-FXII. There is consensus that angioedema attacks in patients with HAE-nC1 do not respond to corticosteroids or antihistamines, even at high doses.[10,33,57,59,60,72,86–88] The drugs and treatment strategies described as effective in HAE-nC1 are largely the same as the ones used in HAE-C1-INH.

On-demand Treatment

C1-INH concentrate: patients with HAE-nC1 have no deficiency of C1-INH, but treatment with C1-INH seems to be effective in many cases, although the effect seems to be more variable than in patients with HAE-C1-INH. In 2016, Bork and colleagues[33] reported the effects of treatment with plasma-derived C1-INH concentrate in 143 facial attacks in 11 patients with HAE-FXII. The mean duration of the attacks was 26.6 hours compared with 64.1 hours for the previous 88 untreated facial attacks. Fifteen laryngeal attacks in 5 patients were treated with plasma-derived C1-INH, resulting in a mean attack duration of 32.7 hours compared with 77.7 hours in 67 untreated attacks. These findings are supported by other reports,[57,59,89,90] but not by all.[10,62,91]

Icatibant: Boccon-Gibod and Bouillet[92] compared self-administered icatibant in patients with HAE-C1-INH (n = 7) and HAE-nC1 (n = 8). They found that icatibant was effective in HAE-nC1. Compared with HAE-C1-INH, the time to first symptom improvement was longer (median 40 minutes, compared with 15 minutes in HAE-C1-INH), and the time to complete symptom resolution was also longer (median 24 hours, compared with 5 hours in HAE-C1-INH). One patient with HAE-C1-INH and 4 patients with HAE-nC1 used a second injection of icatibant to treat their attacks; none of the patients with HAE-C1-INH, but 2 patients with HAE-nC1, used a third injection.[92] Other investigators confirm that icatibant is effective in many patients with HAE-nC1, but most of them also report nonresponders or delayed responses.[57,62,68,93]

Ecallantide has been used successfully by Cronin and Maples[91,94] for repeated on-demand treatment of one patient with HAE-nC1.

Tranexamic acid as on-demand treatment has been shown not to be effective in HAE-C1-INH.[95] In HAE-nC1, treatment effects of intravenous tranexamic acid on demand were reportedly observed in some patients, but the overall effect seemed to be negligible.[62,68]

Fresh frozen plasma has been reported to be effective in an attack of 1 patient with HAE-nC1 not responding to icatibant.[57]

Short-term Prophylaxis

Short-term prophylactic strategies, which are used in HAE-C1-INH to prevent attacks during medical or surgical procedures, have not been studied systematically in HAE-nC1. Similar to HAE-C1-INH, attacks in patients with HAE-FXII can be triggered by mechanical trauma, including dental procedures.[60]

C1-INH concentrate has been used repeatedly for short-term prophylaxis, primarily for deliveries.[57,59,90,96,97] According to the investigators, the treatment was successful; however, there are no data about the frequency of induction of angioedema attacks caused by medical procedures/deliveries in HAE-nC1, so it remains speculation whether the pretreatment with C1-INH concentrate was effective or whether no attack was induced by the procedures. As of now, it is unclear whether and which short-term prophylaxis should be recommended in these patients.

Long-term Prophylaxis

Patients with HAE-nC1 have more disease-free intervals, and their average frequency of attacks is lower compared with patients with HAE-C1-INH.[54,56,57,61,62] Nevertheless, long-term prophylaxis seems to be a common treatment of patients with HAE-nC1.

The therapeutic effects of tranexamic acid in patients with HAE-nC1 seem to be superior to those in patients with HAE-C1-INH, in whom this treatment is unreliable. Several investigators report a good to excellent response to 1.5 to 4 g of tranexamic acid per day in most patients with HAE-nC1. For example, Vitrat-Hincky and colleagues[59] reported a greater than 50% reduction in frequency or severity of attacks in a French cohort of 26 patients with HAE-nC1. Bork and colleagues[33] described a mean reduction in attack frequency of 98.3% in 4 women with HAE-FXII. Deroux and colleagues[56] described 10 patients with HAE-FXII using long-term prophylaxis with tranexamic acid, who showed a reduction of 64% in frequency of attacks compared with the number of attacks before starting prophylactic treatment, and Firinu and colleagues[68] showed a 50% reduction in the number of attacks in 6 patients. Other investigators report failure of long-term prophylaxis with tranexamic acid in parts of their patient population.[10,62]

Recently, Bork and colleagues[33] reported excellent therapeutic responses to progestin in 16 women with HAE-FXII. After discontinuation of estrogen-containing oral contraceptives and switching to progestins (15 desogestrel pill, 1 etonogestrel implant), all women became completely (or nearly) symptom free, and the mean reduction in attack frequency was 99.8% (from 1220 attacks before to 3 attacks under progestins). Similarly, Saule and colleagues[98] showed excellent effects of progestins in 19 women with HAE-nC1, as did 1 Colombian and 2 Spanish groups in 5 patients with HAE-nC1.[57,58,62]

C1-INH concentrate has been reported effective for long-term prophylaxis in HAE-FXII, as described by Deroux and colleagues[56]: Two women were treated with plasma-derived C1-INH concentrate as long-term prophylaxis; however, no further details on the rationale and outcome were presented.

Little information is available on the use of attenuated androgens for long-term prophylaxis in HAE-nC1, possibly because almost all patients are female. Three investigators described danazol to be effective in maintenance doses between 200 mg/wk and 200 mg/d in a total of 5 women.[33,87,99]

REFERENCES

1. Dinkelacker E. Ueber acutes Oedem [Inaugural-Dissertation]. Kiel (Germany): Medicinische Facultät zu Kiel, Kiel; 1882.
2. Quincke H. Über akutes umschriebenes Hautödem. Monatsh Prakt Dermatol 1882;1(5):129–31.
3. Osler W. Hereditary angio-neurotic oedema. Am J Med Sci 1888;95:5.
4. Donaldson VH, Evans RR. A biochemical abnormality in hereditary angioneurotic edema: absence of serum inhibitor of C' 1-esterase. Am J Med 1963;35:37–44.
5. Rosen FS, Pensky J, Donaldson V, et al. Hereditary angioneurotic edema: two genetic variants. Science 1965;148(3672):957–8.
6. Donaldson VH, Ratnoff OD, Dias Da Silva W, et al. Permeability-increasing activity in hereditary angioneurotic edema plasma. II. Mechanism of formation and partial characterization. J Clin Invest 1969;48(4):642–53.
7. Juhlin L, Michaelsson G. Vascular reactions in hereditary angioneurotic edema. Acta Derm Venereol 1969;49(1):20–5.
8. Nussberger J, Cugno M, Amstutz C, et al. Plasma bradykinin in angio-oedema. Lancet 1998;351(9117):1693–7.
9. Binkley KE, Davis A 3rd. Clinical, biochemical, and genetic characterization of a novel estrogen-dependent inherited form of angioedema. J Allergy Clin Immunol 2000;106(3):546–50.
10. Bork K, Barnstedt SE, Koch P, et al. Hereditary angioedema with normal C1-inhibitor activity in women. Lancet 2000;356(9225):213–7.
11. Dewald G, Bork K. Missense mutations in the coagulation factor XII (Hageman factor) gene in hereditary angioedema with normal C1 inhibitor. Biochem Biophys Res Commun 2006;343(4):1286–9.
12. Bork K, Wulff K, Meinke P, et al. A novel mutation in the coagulation factor 12 gene in subjects with hereditary angioedema and normal C1-inhibitor. Clin Immunol 2011;141(1):31–5.
13. Kiss N, Barabas E, Varnai K, et al. Novel duplication in the F12 gene in a patient with recurrent angioedema. Clin Immunol 2013;149(1):142–5.
14. Larsson M, Rayzman V, Nolte MW, et al. A factor XIIa inhibitory antibody provides thromboprotection in extracorporeal circulation without increasing bleeding risk. Sci Transl Med 2014;6(222):222ra217.
15. de Maat S, van Dooremalen S, de Groot PG, et al. A nanobody-based method for tracking factor XII activation in plasma. Thromb Haemost 2013;110(3):458–68.
16. Kannemeier C, Shibamiya A, Nakazawa F, et al. Extracellular RNA constitutes a natural procoagulant cofactor in blood coagulation. Proc Natl Acad Sci U S A 2007;104(15):6388–93.
17. Muller F, Mutch NJ, Schenk WA, et al. Platelet polyphosphates are proinflammatory and procoagulant mediators in vivo. Cell 2009;139(6):1143–56.
18. Oschatz C, Maas C, Lecher B, et al. Mast cells increase vascular permeability by heparin-initiated bradykinin formation in vivo. Immunity 2011;34(2):258–68.
19. Maas C, Govers-Riemslag JW, Bouma B, et al. Misfolded proteins activate factor XII in humans, leading to kallikrein formation without initiating coagulation. J Clin Invest 2008;118(9):3208–18.
20. Zamolodchikov D, Chen ZL, Conti BA, et al. Activation of the factor XII-driven contact system in Alzheimer's disease patient and mouse model plasma. Proc Natl Acad Sci U S A 2015;112(13):4068–73.
21. de Maat S, Maas C. Factor XII: form determines function. J Thromb Haemost 2016;14(8):1498–506.

22. Reshef A, Zanichelli A, Longhurst H, et al. Elevated D-dimers in attacks of hereditary angioedema are not associated with increased thrombotic risk. Allergy 2015; 70(5):506–13.

23. Cugno M, Tedeschi A, Nussberger J. Bradykinin in idiopathic nonhistaminergic angioedema. Clin Exp Allergy 2016;47(1):139–40.

24. Sala-Cunill A, Bjorkqvist J, Senter R, et al. Plasma contact system activation drives anaphylaxis in severe mast cell-mediated allergic reactions. J Allergy Clin Immunol 2015;135(4):1031–43.e1036.

25. van der Linden PW, Hack CE, Eerenberg AJ, et al. Activation of the contact system in insect-sting anaphylaxis: association with the development of angioedema and shock. Blood 1993;82(6):1732–9.

26. Nussberger J, Cugno M, Cicardi M. Bradykinin-mediated angioedema. N Engl J Med 2002;347(8):621–2.

27. Tersteeg C, de Maat S, De Meyer SF, et al. Plasmin cleavage of von Willebrand factor as an emergency bypass for ADAMTS13 deficiency in thrombotic microangiopathy. Circulation 2014;129(12):1320–31.

28. Kaplan AP, Austen KF. A prealbumin activator of prekallikrein. II. Derivation of activators of prekallikrein from active Hageman factor by digestion with plasmin. J Exp Med 1971;133(4):696–712.

29. Myslimi F, Caparros F, Dequatre-Ponchelle N, et al. Orolingual angioedema during or after thrombolysis for cerebral ischemia. Stroke 2016;47(7):1825–30.

30. Hurford R, Rezvani S, Kreimei M, et al. Incidence, predictors and clinical characteristics of orolingual angio-oedema complicating thrombolysis with tissue plasminogen activator for ischaemic stroke. J Neurol Neurosurg Psychiatr 2015; 86(5):520–3.

31. Ewald GA, Eisenberg PR. Plasmin-mediated activation of contact system in response to pharmacological thrombolysis. Circulation 1995;91(1):28–36.

32. Joseph K, Tholanikunnel BG, Wolf B, et al. Deficiency of plasminogen activator inhibitor 2 in plasma of patients with hereditary angioedema with normal C1 inhibitor levels. J Allergy Clin Immunol 2016;137(6):1822–9.e1821.

33. Bork K, Wulff K, Witzke G, et al. Treatment for hereditary angioedema with normal C1-INH and specific mutations in the F12 gene (HAE-FXII). Allergy 2016;72: 320–4.

34. Defendi F, Charignon D, Ghannam A, et al. Enzymatic assays for the diagnosis of bradykinin-dependent angioedema. PLoS One 2013;8(8):e70140.

35. Nielsen EW, Johansen HT, Hogasen K, et al. Activation of the complement, coagulation, fibrinolytic and kallikrein-kinin systems during attacks of hereditary angioedema. Scand J Immunol 1996;44(2):185–92.

36. van Geffen M, Cugno M, Lap P, et al. Alterations of coagulation and fibrinolysis in patients with angioedema due to C1-inhibitor deficiency. Clin Exp Immunol 2012; 167(3):472–8.

37. Cugno M, Hack CE, de Boer JP, et al. Generation of plasmin during acute attacks of hereditary angioedema. J Lab Clin Med 1993;121(1):38–43.

38. van der Linden PW, Hack CE, Struyvenberg A, et al. Controlled insect-sting challenge in 55 patients: correlation between activation of plasminogen and the development of anaphylactic shock. Blood 1993;82(6):1740–8.

39. Germenis AE, Speletas M. Genetics of hereditary angioedema revisited. Clin Rev Allergy Immunol 2016;51(2):170–82.

40. Stieber C, Grumach AS, Cordeiro E, et al. First report of a FXII gene mutation in a Brazilian family with hereditary angio-oedema with normal C1 inhibitor. Br J Dermatol 2015;173(4):1102–4.

41. Moreno AS, Valle SO, Levy S, et al. Coagulation factor XII gene mutation in Brazilian families with hereditary angioedema with normal C1 inhibitor. Int Arch Allergy Immunol 2015;166(2):114–20.

42. Cicardi M, Aberer W, Banerji A, et al. Classification, diagnosis, and approach to treatment for angioedema: consensus report from the Hereditary Angioedema International Working Group. Allergy 2014;69(5):602–16.

43. Cichon S, Martin L, Hennies HC, et al. Increased activity of coagulation factor XII (Hageman factor) causes hereditary angioedema type III. Am J Hum Genet 2006; 79(6):1098–104.

44. Bork K, Kleist R, Hardt J, et al. Kallikrein-kinin system and fibrinolysis in hereditary angioedema due to factor XII gene mutation Thr309Lys. Blood Coagul Fibrinolysis 2009;20(5):325–32.

45. Bjorkqvist J, de Maat S, Lewandrowski U, et al. Defective glycosylation of coagulation factor XII underlies hereditary angioedema type III. J Clin Invest 2015; 125(8):3132–46.

46. de Maat S, de Groot PG, Maas C. Contact system activation on endothelial cells. Semin Thromb Hemost 2014;40(8):887–94.

47. de Maat S, Bjorkqvist J, Suffritti C, et al. Plasmin is a natural trigger for bradykinin production in patients with hereditary angioedema with factor XII mutations. J Allegy Clin Immunol 2016;138(5):1414–23.e1419.

48. Gelincik A, Demir S, Olgac M, et al. Idiopathic angioedema with F12 mutation: is it a new entity? Ann Allergy Asthma Immunol 2015;114(2):154–6.

49. Speletas M, Szilagyi A, Csuka D, et al. F12-46C/T polymorphism as modifier of the clinical phenotype of hereditary angioedema. Allergy 2015;70(12):1661–4.

50. Kanaji T, Okamura T, Osaki K, et al. A common genetic polymorphism (46 C to T substitution) in the 5'-untranslated region of the coagulation factor XII gene is associated with low translation efficiency and decrease in plasma factor XII level. Blood 1998;91(6):2010–4.

51. Kaplan AP, Joseph K. Pathogenic mechanisms of bradykinin mediated diseases: dysregulation of an innate inflammatory pathway. Adv Immunol 2014;121:41–89.

52. Cao H, Hegele RA. DNA polymorphism and mutations in CPN1, including the genomic basis of carboxypeptidase N deficiency. J Hum Genet 2003;48(1):20–2.

53. Dessart P, Defendi F, Humeau H, et al. Distinct conditions support a novel classification for bradykinin-mediated angio-oedema. Dermatology 2015;230(4): 324–31.

54. Bork K, Gul D, Hardt J, et al. Hereditary angioedema with normal C1 inhibitor: clinical symptoms and course. Am J Med 2007;120(11):987–92.

55. Bork K, Wulff K, Witzke G, et al. Hereditary angioedema with normal C1-INH with versus without specific F12 gene mutations. Allergy 2015;70(8):1004–12.

56. Deroux A, Boccon-Gibod I, Fain O, et al. Hereditary angioedema with normal C1 inhibitor and factor XII mutation: a series of 57 patients from the French National Center of Reference for Angioedema. Clin Exp Immunol 2016;185(3):332–7.

57. Pinero-Saavedra M, Gonzalez-Quevedo T, Saenz de San Pedro B, et al. Hereditary angioedema with F12 mutation: clinical features and enzyme polymorphisms in 9 southwestern Spanish families. Ann Allergy Asthma Immunol 2016;117(5): 520–6.

58. Serrano C, Guilarte M, Tella R, et al. Oestrogen-dependent hereditary angio-oedema with normal C1 inhibitor: description of six new cases and review of pathogenic mechanisms and treatment. Allergy 2008;63(6):735–41.

59. Vitrat-Hincky V, Gompel A, Dumestre-Perard C, et al. Type III hereditary angio-oedema: clinical and biological features in a French cohort. Allergy 2010; 65(10):1331–6.
60. Bork K, Wulff K, Hardt J, et al. Hereditary angioedema caused by missense mutations in the factor XII gene: clinical features, trigger factors, and therapy. J Allergy Clin Immunol 2009;124(1):129–34.
61. Bork K. Diagnosis and treatment of hereditary angioedema with normal C1 inhibitor. Allergy Asthma Clin Immunol 2010;6(1):15.
62. Marcos C, Lopez Lera A, Varela S, et al. Clinical, biochemical, and genetic characterization of type III hereditary angioedema in 13 northwest Spanish families. Ann Allergy Asthma Immunol 2012;109(3):195–200.e192.
63. Bork K, Meng G, Staubach P, et al. Hereditary angioedema: new findings concerning symptoms, affected organs, and course. Am J Med 2006;119(3):267–74.
64. Craig TJ, Bernstein JA, Farkas H, et al. Diagnosis and treatment of bradykinin-mediated angioedema: outcomes from an angioedema expert consensus meeting. Int Arch Allergy Immunol 2014;165(2):119–27.
65. Magerl M, Doumoulakis G, Kalkounou I, et al. Characterization of prodromal symptoms in a large population of patients with hereditary angio-oedema. Clin Exp Dermatol 2014;39(3):298–303.
66. Prematta MJ, Kemp JG, Gibbs JG, et al. Frequency, timing, and type of prodromal symptoms associated with hereditary angioedema attacks. Allergy Asthma Proc 2009;30(5):506–11.
67. Reshef A, Prematta MJ, Craig TJ. Signs and symptoms preceding acute attacks of hereditary angioedema: results of three recent surveys. Allergy Asthma Proc 2013;34(3):261–6.
68. Firinu D, Bafunno V, Vecchione G, et al. Characterization of patients with angioedema without wheals: the importance of F12 gene screening. Clin Immunol 2015; 157(2):239–48.
69. Rasmussen ER, de Freitas PV, Bygum A. Urticaria and prodromal symptoms including erythema marginatum in Danish patients with hereditary angioedema. Acta Derm Venereol 2016;96(3):373–6.
70. Zanichelli A, Longhurst HJ, Maurer M, et al. Misdiagnosis trends in patients with hereditary angioedema from the real-world clinical setting. Ann Allergy Asthma Immunol 2016;117(4):394–8.
71. Zanichelli A, Magerl M, Longhurst H, et al. Hereditary angioedema with C1 inhibitor deficiency: delay in diagnosis in Europe. Allergy Asthma Clin Immunol 2013; 9(1):29.
72. Zuraw BL, Bork K, Binkley KE, et al. Hereditary angioedema with normal C1 inhibitor function: consensus of an international expert panel. Allergy Asthma Proc 2012;33(Suppl 1):S145–56.
73. Andersen MF, Longhurst HJ, Rasmussen ER, et al. How not to be misled by disorders mimicking angioedema: a review of pseudoangioedema. Int Arch Allergy Immunol 2016;169(3):163–70.
74. Bas M, Hoffmann TK, Kojda G, et al. ACE-inhibitor induced angioedema. Laryngorhinootologie 2007;86(11):804–8 [quiz: 809–13]. [in German].
75. Ricketti AJ, Cleri DJ, Ramos-Bonner LS, et al. Hereditary angioedema presenting in late middle age after angiotensin-converting enzyme inhibitor treatment. Ann Allergy Asthma Immunol 2007;98(4):397–401.
76. Bork K, Dewald G. Hereditary angioedema type III, angioedema associated with angiotensin II receptor antagonists, and female sex. Am J Med 2004;116(9): 644–5.

77. Sharma VK, Gupta V, Pathak M, et al. An open-label prospective clinical study to assess the efficacy of increasing levocetirizine dose up-to four times in chronic spontaneous urticaria not controlled with standard dose. J Dermatolog Treat 2017. [Epub ahead of print].

78. Staevska M, Popov TA, Kralimarkova T, et al. The effectiveness of levocetirizine and desloratadine in up to 4 times conventional doses in difficult-to-treat urticaria. J Allergy Clin Immunol 2010;125(3):676–82.

79. Azofra J, Diaz C, Antepara I, et al. Positive response to omalizumab in patients with acquired idiopathic nonhistaminergic angioedema. Ann Allergy Asthma Immunol 2015;114(5):418–9.e411.

80. Faisant C, Du Thanh A, Mansard C, et al. Idiopathic non-histaminergic angioedema: successful treatment with omalizumab in five patients. J Clin Immunol 2016;37:80–4.

81. Munoz JP, Casado AF, Taboada AC, et al. Successful treatment of refractory idiopathic angio-oedema with omalizumab: review of the literature and function of IgE in angio-oedema. Clin Exp Dermatol 2016;41(4):399–402.

82. Ozturk AB, Kocaturk E. Omalizumab in recurring larynx angioedema: a case report. Asia Pac Allergy 2014;4(2):129–30.

83. Sands MF, Blume JW, Schwartz SA. Successful treatment of 3 patients with recurrent idiopathic angioedema with omalizumab. J Allergy Clin Immunol 2007;120(4):979–81.

84. Staubach P, Metz M, Chapman-Rothe N, et al. Effect of omalizumab on angioedema in H1 -antihistamine-resistant chronic spontaneous urticaria patients: results from X-ACT, a randomized controlled trial. Allergy 2016;71(8):1135–44.

85. von Websky A, Reich K, Steinkraus V, et al. Complete remission of severe chronic recurrent angioedema of unknown cause with omalizumab. J Dtsch Dermatol Ges 2013;11(7):677–8.

86. Bell CG, Kwan E, Nolan RC, et al. First molecular confirmation of an Australian case of type III hereditary angioedema. Pathology 2008;40(1):82–3.

87. Herrmann G, Schneider L, Krieg T, et al. Efficacy of danazol treatment in a patient with the new variant of hereditary angio-oedema (HAE III). Br J Dermatol 2004;150(1):157–8.

88. Prieto A, Tornero P, Rubio M, et al. Missense mutation Thr309Lys in the coagulation factor XII gene in a Spanish family with hereditary angioedema type III. Allergy 2009;64(2):284–6.

89. Deroux A, Vilgrain I, Dumestre-Perard C, et al. Towards a specific marker for acute bradykinin-mediated angioedema attacks: a literature review. Eur J Dermatol 2015;25(4):290–5.

90. Bouillet L, Ponard D, Rousset H, et al. A case of hereditary angio-oedema type III presenting with C1-inhibitor cleavage and a missense mutation in the F12 gene. Br J Dermatol 2007;156(5):1063–5.

91. Cronin JA, Maples KM. Treatment of an acute attack of type III hereditary angioedema with ecallantide. Ann Allergy Asthma Immunol 2012;108(1):61–2.

92. Boccon-Gibod I, Bouillet L. Safety and efficacy of icatibant self-administration for acute hereditary angioedema. Clin Exp Immunol 2012;168(3):303–7.

93. Bouillet L, Boccon-Gibod I, Ponard D, et al. Bradykinin receptor 2 antagonist (icatibant) for hereditary angioedema type III attacks. Ann Allergy Asthma Immunol 2009;103(5):448.

94. Cronin JA, Minto HB, Maples KM. Re: successful management of hereditary angioedema with normal C1-INH (type III HAE) when using on-demand ecallantide. J Allergy Clin Immunol Pract 2014;2(2):239.

95. Zanichelli A, Mansi M, Azin GM, et al. Efficacy of on-demand treatment in reducing morbidity in patients with hereditary angioedema due to C1 inhibitor deficiency. Allergy 2015;70(12):1553–8.

96. Picone O, Donnadieu AC, Brivet FG, et al. Obstetrical complications and outcome in two families with hereditary angioedema due to mutation in the F12 gene. Obstet Gynecol Int 2010;2010:957507.

97. Yu SK, Callum J, Alam A. C1-esterase inhibitor for short-term prophylaxis in a patient with hereditary angioedema with normal C1 inhibitor function. J Clin Anesth 2016;35:488–91.

98. Saule C, Boccon-Gibod I, Fain O, et al. Benefits of progestin contraception in non-allergic angioedema. Clin Exp Allergy 2013;43(4):475–82.

99. Martin L, Degenne D, Toutain A, et al. Hereditary angioedema type III: an additional French pedigree with autosomal dominant transmission. J Allergy Clin Immunol 2001;107(4):747–8.

Emerging Therapies in Hereditary Angioedema

Meng Chen, MD*, Marc A. Riedl, MD, MS

KEYWORDS

- Angioedema • Emerging therapies • C1 esterase inhibitor • Bradykinin • Kallikrein
- Factor XII

KEY POINTS

- Although significant therapeutic progress has been made in hereditary angioedema (HAE), current treatments are still limited by access, cost, and side effects.
- Multiple new therapies are being investigated for the treatment of HAE due to C1 esterase inhibitor deficiency.
- Novel mechanisms of action and drug delivery include subcutaneous complement component 1 esterase inhibitor (C1INH) concentrates, a monoclonal antibody inhibitor of kallikrein, oral kallikrein inhibitors, RNA-targeted antisense against prekallikrein, RNA interference drugs against factor XII, monoclonal antibody inhibitor of factor XIIa, and gene therapy.
- Studies are ongoing to expand the number of drugs available for pediatric patients with HAE due to C1 esterase inhibitor deficiency.

INTRODUCTION

Angioedema occurs due to the transient movement of fluid from the vasculature into the interstitial space leading to subcutaneous (SC) or submucosal swelling, which can have life-threatening consequences. Current evidence suggests that most angioedema conditions can be grouped into 2 categories: histamine-mediated or bradykinin-mediated angioedema. Although effective therapies for histamine-mediated angioedema have existed for decades, effective therapies for bradykinin-mediated angioedema have only more recently been developed, studied rigorously, and approved by regulatory agencies. As such, the treatment options for hereditary angioedema (HAE) have increased substantially over the last decade.

In the United States, therapy for HAE angioedema attacks was largely supportive a decade ago. Currently, 4 effective HAE-specific acute treatment options are available.[1] In addition, advances in HAE-specific prophylactic treatment have been

Division of Rheumatology, Department of Medicine, Allergy & Immunology, University of California San Diego, 8899 University City Lane, Suite 230, San Diego, CA 92122, USA
* Corresponding author.
E-mail address: mec079@ucsd.edu

Immunol Allergy Clin N Am 37 (2017) 585–595
http://dx.doi.org/10.1016/j.iac.2017.03.003   **immunology.theclinics.com**
0889-8561/17/© 2017 Elsevier Inc. All rights reserved.

realized and continue to evolve. This article primarily focuses on emerging treatments for bradykinin-mediated angioedema, specifically HAE due to complement component 1 esterase inhibitor (C1INH) deficiency, because most recent research and therapeutic development has focused on improved prevention of HAE symptoms. To provide context for therapeutic strategies, this article provides a cursory review of the pathophysiology of angioedema (**Fig. 1**).

HISTAMINERGIC VERSUS BRADYKININ PATHWAYS

As detailed in other articles of this issue, angioedema is generally caused by 1 of 2 mechanisms: through a mast cell–mediated pathway (histaminergic angioedema) or through a nonhistaminergic pathway. Current evidence strongly supports bradykinin as the predominant mediator responsible for nonhistaminergic forms of angioedema. Clinically distinguishing between these 2 pathways is paramount in selecting the appropriate agents for both acute and preventative treatment because these 2 categories respond to completely different classes of medications.

Histaminergic angioedema is mediated by mast cell activation with release of histamine, leukotrienes, and other mast cell–associated mediators. This form of angioedema is often accompanied by urticaria or pruritus and is seen in immunoglobulin (Ig)-E–mediated allergic reactions due to food, medication, or venom allergy, though a substantial portion of recurrent histaminergic angioedema is idiopathic in nature.

Nonhistaminergic angioedema seems to be primarily mediated by bradykinin dysregulation wherein symptoms result from the overproduction of bradykinin, which causes vasodilatation and vascular permeability by binding to the bradykinin B2 receptor on endothelial cells.[2] Bradykinin is generated through the activation of the kallikrein-kinin (contact) system, although the precise mechanisms are still poorly understood. Angioedema episodes are believed to be initiated by activation of the contact system, prekallikrein and factor XII, forming factor XIIa and kallikrein. Bradykinin is formed by cleavage of high molecular weight kininogen by plasma kallikrein. C1INH is a serine protease that inhibits proteases involved in this pathway. HAE due to C1INH

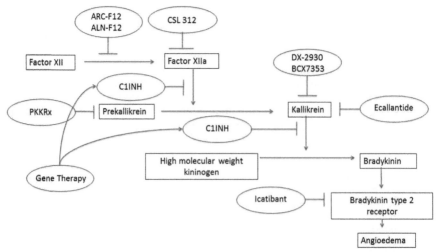

Fig. 1. Pathogenesis of bradykinin-mediated angioedema with targets for existing and developing therapies. C1INH, complement component 1 inhibitor.

deficiency occurs with mutations in the SERPING1 gene. Bradykinin-mediated angioedema can be due to HAE with C1INH deficiency or with normal C1INH, acquired C1INH deficiency, or angiotensin-converting enzyme (ACE) inhibitor–induced angioedema. HAE is classically diagnosed through C1INH deficiency, though a subset of patients who behave similarly to patients with classic HAE have normal levels of C1INH.

Treatment of Histamine Versus Bradykinin-Mediated Angioedema

Historically, histamine-mediated angioedema has been more successfully managed given the availability of effective medications for mast cell–mediated conditions (eg, antihistamines, corticosteroids, epinephrine, omalizumab), as well as health care providers' familiarity with the allergic pathway as a cause of angioedema symptoms. Most treatment deficits and unmet need have involved the bradykinin-mediated angioedema conditions, most prominently HAE. Thus, almost all recent research and development efforts in angioedema therapy have focused on the bradykinin pathway. Recent clinical work in histamine-mediated angioedema has largely confirmed the efficacy of existing histamine-targeted therapies.[3,4] As such, the remainder of this article focuses on therapeutic development efforts in bradykinin-mediated angioedema.

RECENT DEVELOPMENTS IN HEREDITARY ANGIOEDEMA THERAPY
Hereditary Angioedema Therapy for Pediatrics

Pediatric HAE is currently an area of unmet need requiring additional therapeutic advances. Many HAE patients will experience their first attack in childhood and pediatric patients currently have limited treatment options due to a lack of pediatric efficacy and safety data with most HAE medications. Plasma-derived C1INH concentrate (Berinert) is to date the only treatment for acute attacks in HAE patients younger than 12 years approved by the US Food and Drug Administration (FDA). There are currently no FDA-approved drugs for long-term prophylaxis in pediatric HAE patients. Pediatric patients may often be treated with HAE-specific medications in an off label approach with limited controlled data to guide these decisions.[5] Data from uncontrolled trials support the use of C1INH concentrate (Cinryze) and tranexamic acid for prophylaxis, and icatibant for on demand treatment in children. Data from uncontrolled trials suggests the efficacy of danazol prophylaxis for children but use is not recommended given the numerous potentially serious adverse effects. Several clinical trials are ongoing to evaluate the efficacy of HAE-specific medications for the pediatric population.

Clinical trials

A phase 2, multicenter, open-label study was conducted to investigate the safety and efficacy of ecallantide in the treatment of children and adolescents experiencing an acute HAE attack (NCT01832896). Subjects between the ages of 2 and 15 years of age were included in the study. Ecallantide is currently FDA-approved for patients 12 years and older. Pediatric patients experiencing an angioedema attack were treated with varying SC doses depending on weight. The estimated primary completion date was July 2015, though no results have been published.

Recombinant C1INH (Ruconest) is currently being studied in a phase 2, open-label, single-arm study to evaluate the safety, immunogenicity, and pharmacology in the treatment of acute HAE attacks in children between the ages of 2 and 13 years (NCT01359969). Recombinant C1INH is currently FDA-approved for adolescents and adults for treatment of acute attacks. Within the study, subjects experiencing an acute HAE attack who weigh less than 84 kg will receive 50units/kg of Ruconest in a 1-time intravenous (IV) injection; subjects who weigh more than 84 kg will receive

4200 units. The estimated date of completion for collection of primary data is December 2017.

A phase 3, multicenter, open-label, nonrandomized study is ongoing to assess the safety and pharmacology of icatibant in children older than 2 years and adolescents younger than 18 years in the treatment of acute HAE attacks (NCT01386658). Icatibant is currently FDA-approved for adults 18 years and older. Pediatric subjects experiencing an acute HAE attack will receive a single dose of icatibant 0.4 mg/kg SC up to a maximal dose of 30 mg and will be followed for 90 days. The estimated study completion date is September 2017.

A phase 3, multicenter, randomized, single-blinded, dose-ranging, crossover study is in progress to evaluate the safety and efficacy of Cinryze for long-term HAE prophylaxis in children between the ages of 6 and 11 years (NCT02052141). This study will evaluate the relative efficacy of Cinryze 500 units or 1000 units IV every 3 to 4 days to prevent angioedema attacks in a 12-week treatment period. Subjects will receive the alternate dose the following 12 weeks. The estimated completion of primary data collection is in May 2017.

EMERGING THERAPIES FOR LONG-TERM PROPHYLAXIS
Treatments in Human Studies

Complement component 1 esterase inhibitor concentrates
Currently, 3 IV C1INH concentrates are available for the treatment of HAE with 1 product licensed by the FDA for long-term prophylactic therapy. However, frequently, patients have limited or difficult vascular access, which complicates use of repeated IV medication. In some cases, the placement of a long-term catheter is required for therapy, which poses additional risks, such as infection and thrombosis. A SC route of administration would obviate these challenges and provide an additional prophylactic option for patients.

Subcutaneous complement component 1 esterase inhibitor Two SC plasma-derived C1INH concentrates are currently being studied for long-term prevention of HAE attacks.

Early studies conducted by CSL Behring with SC C1INH demonstrated the SC drug to be well-tolerated, with sufficient bioavailability to be a viable treatment option. The PASSION study was a prospective, randomized, open-label study with subjects receiving Berinert either via IV or SC infusion using 1000 U in 20 mL of solution.[6] Administration of the IV solution occurred over 3 minutes, whereas the SC administration occurred over 15 minutes at 2 separate abdominal sites (500 U at each site).

The investigators reported 15 out of 24 subjects (62.5%) receiving the SC formulation had a total of 32 adverse events as compared with 7 of the 24 subjects (29.2%) who received the IV administration with a total of 14 adverse events. All adverse events reported in the IV group were reported unlikely or not caused by the drug, whereas 23 of the 32 adverse events in the SC group were possibly or probably related to the drug. All of the reactions in the SC group were classified as mild, consisting predominantly of irritation and swelling at the infusion site. SC administration of Berinert resulted in 39.7% bioavailability compared with IV administration. C1INH functional levels were lower after SC as compared with IV administration but the mean half-life of C1INH was longer with SC compared with IV administration (120 hours vs 62 hours). Although SC administration resulted in reduced bioavailability, pharmacodynamic studies revealed this level could exert an appreciable increase in C4 antigen and a decrease in cleaved high molecular weight kininogen (ClHK).

The COMPACT phase II study was an open-label, dose-ranging, crossover study examining the pharmacology and safety of an SC C1INH, CSL830.[7] Eighteen subjects first received a single dose of Berinert 20U/kg IV within 2 to 7 days of receiving CSL830. The subjects then received twice weekly SC injections of CSL830, a highly concentrated, volume-reduced C1INH, for 4 weeks followed by a washout of 4 weeks, and then received a different concentration of CSL830 for another 4 weeks. Subjects received 2 of 3 doses (1500, 3000, or 6000 IU). The trough functional C1INH activity level and C4 antigen level were found to increase in a dose-dependent manner with CSL830 treatment. Subjects in the 3000 and 6000 IU dose groups reached and maintained a C1INH activity level greater than 40% of normal, postulated as a level adequate to prevent angioedema attacks. CSL830 also demonstrated a more consistent level of exposure compared with IV administration with a lower peak-to-trough ratio. Safety data for CSL830 was reassuring with no serious related adverse events, deaths, or thromboembolic events. CSL830 was generally well-tolerated; the most common adverse event was local pain and swelling at the infusion site. Moderate site swelling was reported in 5 of 12 subjects receiving the 6000 IU dose compared with 1 of 12 subjects in the 3000 IU dose group and 2 of 12 subjects in the 1500 IU dose group. Seven subjects experienced 29 angioedema-related events, with 11 events occurring during weeks of drug exposure and 18 events occurring outside of drug exposure periods. During the drug exposure period, 2 subjects in the 1500 IU and 2 subjects in the 3000 IU groups experienced all of the attacks, whereas 0 subjects in the 6000 IU groups had an attack.

A phase III double-blinded, randomized, placebo-controlled, crossover study was recently completed to assess the efficacy of SC C1INH compared with placebo in the prevention of HAE angioedema attacks.[8] Ninety subjects were randomized in a 1:1:1:1 fashion to 1of 4 treatment arms. Each treatment arm included 2 16-week treatment periods. Subjects received either 40IU/kg or 60IU/kg of CSL830 in twice weekly SC injections followed by placebo, or vice versa. Seventy-nine of 90 subjects completed the study. The primary endpoint was time-normalized number of HAE attacks. Both doses of the study drug significantly reduced the number of HAE attacks compared with placebo with a P value of less than .001. The lower dose group had a mean difference of −2.42 attacks per month (95% CI −3.38 to −1.46) representing an 89% median reduction. The higher dose group had a mean difference of −3.51 attacks per month (95% CI −4.21 to −2.81) representing a 95% median reduction. Secondary endpoints included response rate (defined as subjects with at least a 50% reduction in time-normalized number of HAE attacks as compared with placebo), and time-normalized number of rescue medications required, as well as adverse events. The lower dose group had a 76% response rate (95% CI 62–87) and the higher dose group had a 90% response rate (95% CI 77–96). The number of rescue medications used in the placebo group was 5.55 uses per month as compared with 1.13 in the lower dose group, and 3.89 in the placebo group as compared with 0.32 in the higher dose group. Consistent with previous trials, most adverse events were mild injection site reactions. These study data have been submitted to the FDA for review.

A SC formulation of the plasma-derived C1INH concentrate, Cinryze, is being developed for prophylaxis of HAE attacks. In 2010, a phase II, open-label, multiple-dose study evaluated the safety and pharmacology of SC versus IV administration of Cinryze (NCT01095497). Results from clinicaltrials.gov show 26 subjects first received 1000 units of IV Cinryze twice weekly for 18 days followed by a 14-day washout period, and then received 1 of 2 doses of SC Cinryze. Subjects either received 1000 units of Cinryze SC twice weekly for 2 weeks or 2000 units of Cinryze SC twice weekly for 2 weeks. One subject in the lower dose SC group withdrew from the study. Twelve out of 26 subjects in the IV group reported adverse events, 1 of whom reported an injection site reaction. Ten of the 13 subjects in the lower dose SC group and 11 of 12 in the higher dose SC group reported adverse events, all of which were injection site reactions. There were no serious adverse events.

A phase II, open-label, multiple-dose study evaluated the safety and pharmacology of Cinryze with recombinant human hyaluronidase (rHuPH20) in HAE subjects in 2011 (NCT01426763). The results on clinicaltrials.gov show 12 subjects received either 1000 units of Cinryze with 20,000 units of rHuPH20 or 2000 units of Cinryze with 40,000 units of rHuPH20 twice weekly for 2 weeks. Eleven of 12 subjects experienced adverse events, which were largely local site reactions manifested with erythema, swelling, and/or pain. Pharmacology results were not reported.

A phase II, randomized, double-blinded, multicenter, dose-ranging, crossover study examined the safety and efficacy of SC Cinryze with rHuPH20 in 2012.[9] Subjects received either 1000 units of Cinryze with 24,000 units of rHuPH20 or 2000 units of Cinryze with 48,000 units of rHuPH20 as a single 20 mL SC injection twice weekly for 8 weeks. The primary outcome measure was normalized number of angioedema attacks during the treatment period. Subjects in the lower dose treatment group had a normalized number of angioedema attacks of 1.58 (95% CI 0.88–2.29) as compared with 0.97 (0.41–1.53) in the higher dose treatment group with a P value of .0523. Secondary outcome measures showed a statistically significant lower severity of attacks and lower number of attacks that required acute treatment in the higher dose treatment group. There were no serious adverse events in either group; almost all subjects experienced local injection site reactions. Of note, 45% of subjects had detectable non-neutralizing antibodies to rHuPH20. None of the antibodies to rHuPH20 were associated with adverse effects but the study was terminated early as a precaution. The pharmacokinetic data were variable, but there appeared to be no significant bioavailability advantage with the use of hyaluronidase.

Based on this study data, a phase III, randomized, double-blind, placebo-controlled, 2-period, 3-sequence, partial crossover study to evaluate the safety and efficacy of a SC liquid formulation of C1INH without the use of recombinant human hyaluronidase is currently ongoing (NCT02584959). Target completion of primary data collection is in December 2017.

Recombinant human C1INH Recombinant human C1INH (rhC1INH) is being investigated for long-term prophylaxis for HAE. Recently, a phase II, randomized, double-blind, placebo-controlled trial was completed with data presented at the ACAAI 2016 meeting.[10] Subjects 13 years and older were randomized to 3 separate 4-week treatment periods separated by a 1 week washout period. Subjects were assigned to 1 of 6 treatment sequences with all arms, including treatment periods with rhC1INH 50IU/kg IV twice weekly, rhC1INH 50IU/kg IV once weekly plus saline IV once weekly, and saline IV twice weekly. Study results demonstrated that IV rhC1INH treatment significantly reduced the number of HAE attacks as compared with placebo. Subjects in the 50IU/kg twice weekly arm experienced a mean of 2.7 attacks over the 4-week period and subjects in the 50IU/kg once weekly arm experienced a mean of 4.4 attacks over 4 weeks compared with 7.2 attacks over 4 weeks in the placebo arm ($P<.0001$ and $P<.0004$, respectively). A clinical response (defined as $\geq 50\%$ reduction in number of HAE attacks) was observed in 95.7% of subjects during the 50IU/kg twice weekly period and 56.5% of subjects during the 50IU/kg once weekly period. Overall, the drug was well-tolerated with no drug-related serious adverse events reported.

Monoclonal antibody inhibitor of kallikrein

Lanadelumab (DX2930 or SHP643) A fully human monoclonal antibody inhibitor of plasma kallikrein was developed by Dyax, now part of Shire. Initially known as DX2930, the drug has more recently been designated as SHP643 and named lanadelumab. A phase 1, single-center, double-blinded, randomized study with 32 subjects studied SC administration in 4 sequential dose cohorts using 0.1, 0.3, 1.0 or 3.0 mg/kg of DX2930. Pharmacokinetic and pharmacodynamic studies revealed a dose-dependent and time-dependent inhibition of kallikrein with a long-acting effect favorable for long-term prophylaxis. No serious adverse events were observed.[11] Subsequently, a phase 1b study has been completed with 37 subjects randomized to 4 doses of DX2930 (30, 100, 300, or 400 mg) or placebo.[12] The 300 mg treatment arm demonstrated a 100% reduction in HAE attacks as compared with placebo ($P<.0001$) and the 400 mg arm showed a 88% reduction HAE attacks ($P = .05$) in the primary efficacy assessment period from days 8 to 50. Cohort numbers were small but 4 out of 4 subjects in the 300 mg arm were attack-free during this assessment period, and 9 out of 11 subjects in the 400 mg arm were attack-free as compared with 3 out of 11 subjects in the placebo arm ($P = .026$ and $P = .030$, respectively). No serious adverse events or safety signals were identified in the study.

Currently, a phase III, multicenter, randomized, double-blinded, placebo-controlled clinical trial of lanadelumab for the long-term prevention of HAE attacks is underway (NCT02586805). The study will investigate the efficacy and safety of SC doses of lanadelumab at 150 mg every 4 weeks, 300 mg every 2 weeks, and 300 mg every 4 weeks compared with placebo. Completion of data collection for the primary outcome is expected in 2017.

Oral kallikrein inhibitors

Development of effective and safe oral medications for prophylaxis of HAE attacks would provide a potentially important alternative to injected or infused medications. The current oral options include antifibrinolytics, which lack relative efficacy and require multiple daily dosing, and attenuated androgens, which are complicated by significant long-term adverse effects for many patients. Development of oral small molecule plasma kallikrein inhibitors is being pursued by BioCryst and KalVista.

Avoralstat (BCX4161) A first-generation oral small molecule kallikrein inhibitor, Avoralstat (BCX4161) (NCT02670720), has been studied with preclinical, phase I, and phase II study data supporting safety and efficacy. However, a recently completed placebo-controlled phase III study failed to show a significant reduction in the frequency of HAE attacks for the active drug versus placebo. Subjects (110) were randomized to treatment with avoralstat (500 mg or 300 mg) or placebo 3 times daily for 12 weeks. No statistically significant differences were observed in the mean attack rate with either treatment arm as compared with placebo (mean attack rate of 0.63 per week in the 500 mg arm, 0.71 per week in the 300 mg arm, and 0.61 per week in the placebo arm).[13] Pharmacokinetic data collected during the trial indicated that drug exposure was suboptimal within treated subjects due to low and variable bioavailability. Avoralstat required a 3 times daily dosing regimen during the phase III study. Avoralstat clinical development has been halted based on these findings.

BCX7353 A second generation kallikrein inhibitor, BCX7353, is currently in development. Results from a phase I clinical trial with 122 healthy subjects demonstrated

BCX7353 to be safe and well-tolerated. There were no reported serious adverse events, and 89% of adverse events were mild. The remaining adverse events were moderate and included nausea, vomiting, hay fever, and self-limited diarrhea. Of subjects who received the drug for at least 7 days, 5% developed a self-limited skin rash.[14] Pharmacodynamic and pharmacokinetic studies supported a once-daily dosing regimen, unlike its predecessor Avoralstat. Part 1 of a phase II, randomized, double-blinded, placebo-controlled, dose-ranging, parallel-group study to evaluate the efficacy, safety, and pharmacologic properties of BCX7353 is currently underway (NCT02870972). Twenty-four subjects will be randomized to BCX7353 350 mg once daily or placebo daily for 4 weeks. If an interim analysis supports efficacy, part 2 of this trial will include randomization to additional doses (250 mg daily and 125 mg daily) to assess for dose responsiveness. Target completion of primary outcome data collection is in April 2017.[15]

KVD818 KVD818, an oral plasma kallikrein inhibitor, is currently in phase I human clinical studies; no study data on the molecule have been published to date.[16]

Antisense targeting prekallikrein
Ionis PKKRx Ionis Pharmaceuticals is developing antisense therapy for HAE prophylaxis, targeting the reduction of prekallikrein.[17,18] A phase 1, blinded, placebo-controlled, dose-escalation clinical trial completed in 2015 demonstrated a 95% reduction in prekallikrein in healthy volunteers. The drug was well-tolerated and safe in both single and multiple-dose arms. The company has indicated plans to move forward with this clinical development program for the prevention of HAE attacks.

Treatments in Preclinical Studies

Factor XII
Factor XII is cleaved into factor XIIa and is involved in the initiation of contact system activation that ultimately leads to bradykinin production and increased vascular permeability. C1INH normally inhibits this signaling cascade but, in the deficient state, excess factor XII activation seems to be a critical factor for HAE symptoms, thus making it an attractive target for preventative therapy.

ALN-F12 Alnylam Pharmaceuticals is developing a RNA interference (RNAi) drug (ALN-F12) to knockdown factor XII as a prophylactic treatment of HAE. Preclinical data was presented at the 2016 American Academy of Allergy, Asthma, and Immunology (AAAAI) annual meeting.[19,20] ALN-F12 inhibits factor XII gene expression through degradation of factor XII mRNA. The drug is administered SC, with preliminary studies completed in mice and nonhuman primates. Animal studies have demonstrated a significant reduction of factor XII mRNA with drug treatment and a dose-dependent reduction of vascular permeability in both ACE inhibitor–induced and mustard oil–induced mouse models of bradykinin-induced vascular permeability. In cynomolgus monkeys, a single dose of ALN-F12 exhibited a dose-dependent decrease in plasma factor XII that was maintained for 2 months. The highest dose studied was 3 mg/kg with a greater than 85% reduction in plasma factor XII levels at 1 month and more than a 75% reduction in plasma factor XII levels at 2 months.

ARC-F12 Arrowhead Research Corporation is developing an RNAi drug against factor XII (ARC-F12).[21,22] Studies in rat models have shown greater than 90% knockdown of factor XII with monthly injections of 4 mg/kg of ARC-F12. Treatment with ARC-F12 significantly decreased paw swelling in a rat model of carrageenan-induced paw edema.

Monoclonal antibody antifactor XIIa A recombinant, fully human, monoclonal antibody-blocking factor XIIa (CSL 312) is in preclinical development. Preliminary data were presented at the AAAAI conference in February 2015.[23] The initial compound, 3F7, selected from a human phage display antibody library, was shown to be a potent and specific inhibitor of factor XIIa in enzymatic studies with binding capability to rabbit, mouse, and human-activated factor XII. Murine models have demonstrated attenuation of contact-system–induced skin edema with 3F7 administration. Subsequently, a C1INH deficient mouse model has demonstrated the ability of 3F7 to modulate captopril-induced vascular permeability. CSL312 is a 3F7-variant that has improved affinity and potency.

Gene therapy

Gene therapy for HAE due to C1INH deficiency remains an attractive conceptual treatment approach given the curative potential. Viral vector-based gene replacement and gene editing techniques are methods of considerable interest. Early preclinical work at Weill Medical College of Cornell School of Medicine in the department of Genetics (National Institutes of Health project number 1R03AI122040–01) has been instrumental in the development of adeno-associated virus (AAV) gene therapy in HAE. Adverum Biotechnologies is actively advancing clinical development of this technology: ADVM-053 is an AAV-based gene transfer vector aimed at increasing plasma C1INH levels via C1INH gene therapy, with human studies planned for 2017. If successful, such therapy could prevent attacks, as well as reduce the burden of repeated medication use.

ACUTE THERAPY: CONCEPTUAL
Oral Kallikrein Inhibitor

As discussed, oral kallikrein inhibitors are currently in development for long-term prophylaxis. Pharmacokinetic studies have suggested a maximal plasma drug level within 2 to 5 hours for BCX7353 (and previously 1 to 2 hours for failed drug Avoralstat). This has raised consideration of oral kallikrein inhibitor use for acute therapy to treat HAE attacks. Oral on-demand therapy would provide HAE patients with a convenient option and provide greater treatment flexibility in their daily lives because all current acute therapies require IV or SC injections. Enthusiasm for investigating the use of oral kallikrein inhibitors in acute attacks has been tempered somewhat by the potential challenges of administration and absorption for attacks involving the mouth, throat, and gastrointestinal tract. In addition, the pharmacokinetic and pharmacodynamic parameters may not provide rapid symptom relief comparable to that seen with currently approved acute HAE medications. Phase I pharmacokinetic studies of BCX7353 showed that absorption was slowed in the setting of food consumption, which could be an additional concern. Thus, the clinical utility of an oral acute treatment approach for HAE remains undefined until future studies provide additional data.

FUTURE CONSIDERATIONS AND SUMMARY

The landscape of therapeutic options for patients with bradykinin-mediated angioedema has changed dramatically in the last decade. Ongoing research promises even greater change in the foreseeable future. Given the economic and psychosocial burdens for patients living with angioedema, effective therapies with novel mechanisms will offer more choices for patients and physicians, as well provide greater flexibility in routes of administration. Ultimately, gene therapy strategies may offer a more definitive durable treatment, obviating chronic repeated medication use, though the safety and tolerability of such approaches remains largely unknown.

REFERENCES

1. Bork K. A decade of change: recent developments in pharmacotherapy of hereditary angioedema (HAE). Clin Rev Allergy Immunol 2016;51:183–92.
2. Zuraw BL, Christiansen SC. HAE pathophysiology and underlying mechanisms. Clin Rev Allergy Immunol 2016;51:216–29.
3. von Websky A, Reich K, Steinkraus V, et al. Complete remission of severe chronic recurrent angioedema of unknown cause with omalizumab. J Dtsch Dermatol Ges 2013;11:677–8, 46.
4. Sands MF, Blume JW, Schwartz SA. Successful treatment of 3 patients with recurrent idiopathic angioedema with omalizumab. J Allergy Clin Immunol 2007;120: 979–81.
5. Frank MM, Zuraw B, Banerji A, et al, US hereditary angioedema association medical advisory board. Management of children with hereditary angioedema due to C1 inhibitor deficiency. Pediatrics 2016;138(5).
6. Martinez-Saguer I, Cicardi M, Suffritti C, et al. Pharmacokinetics of plasma-derived C1-INH after SC versus intravenous (IV) administration in subjects with mild or moderate hereditary angioedema: the PASSION study. Transfusion 2014;54(6):1552–61.
7. Zuraw BL, Cicardi M, Longhurst HJ, et al. Phase II study results of a replacement therapy for hereditary angioedema with subcutaneous C1-inhibitor concentrate. Allergy 2015;70(10):1319–28.
8. Longhurst H, Cicardi M, Craig T, et al. Prevention of hereditary angioedema attacks with a subcutaneous C1 inhibitor. N Engl J Med 2017;23;376(12):1131–40.
9. Riedl MA, Lumry WR, Li HH, et al. Subcutaneous administration of human C1 inhibitor with recombinant human hyaluronidase in patients with hereditary angioedema. Allergy Asthma Proc 2016;37:489–500.
10. Riedl MA, Panovska VG, Moldovan D, et al. Randomized, double-blind placebo-controlled trial of recombinant human C1 inhibitor for prophylaxis of hereditary angioedema attacks. San Francisco (CA): ACAAI; 2017.
11. Chyung Y, Vince B, Iarrobino R, et al. A phase 1 study investigating DX-2930 in healthy subjects. Ann Allergy Asthma Immunol 2014;113(4):460–6.e2.
12. Banerji A, Busse P, Shennak M, et al. Inhibiting Plasma Kallikrein for Hereditary Angioedema Prophylaxis. N Engl J Med 2017;376(8):717–28.
13. Available at: http://investor.shareholder.com/biocryst/releasedetail.cfm?ReleaseID=953694. Accessed October 17, 2016.
14. Available at: https://globenewswire.com/news-release/2016/08/11/863629/0/en/BioCryst-Announces-Initiation-of-the-APeX-1-Clinical-Trial-of-BCX7353-for-Hereditary-Angioedema.html. Accessed October 17, 2016.
15. Available at: http://www.biocryst.com/bcx_4161. Accessed October 17, 2016.
16. Available at: http://www.kalvista.com/hae.html. Accessed October 17, 2016.
17. Bhattacharjee G, Revenko AS, Crosby JR, et al. Inhibition of vascular permeability by antisense-mediated inhibition of plasma kallikrein and coagulation factor 12. Nucleic Acid Ther 2013;23:175–87.
18. Revenko AS, Gao D, Crosby JR, et al. Selective depletion of plasma prekallikrein or coagulation factor XII inhibits thrombosis in mice without increased risk of bleeding. Blood 2011;118:5302–11.
19. Liu J, Qin J, Castoreno A, et al. An investigational RNAi therapeutic targeting factor XII (ALN-F12) for the treatment of hereditary angioedema. Los Angeles (CA): AAAAI; 2016. Poster.

20. Available at: http://www.alnylam.com/capella/presentations/new-program-aln-f12/. Accessed October 17, 2016.
21. Melquist S, Wakefield D, Hamilton H, et al. Targeting factor 12 (F12) with a novel RNAi delivery platform as a prophylactic treatment for hereditary angioedema (HAE). Los Angeles (CA): AAAAI; 2016. Poster.
22. Available at: http://arrowheadpharma.com/pipeline/. Accessed October 17, 2016.
23. Cao Z, Biondo M, Rayzman V, et al. Development and characterization of an anti-FXIIa monoclonal antibody for the treatment of hereditary angioedema. Houston (TX): AAAAI; 2015.

Burden of Illness and Quality-of-Life Measures in Angioedema Conditions

Teresa Caballero, MD, PhD[a,b,*], Nieves Prior, MD, PhD[c]

KEYWORDS

- Angioedema • Quality of life • Depression • Anxiety • Burden
- Health-related quality of life • Patient-reported outcomes

KEY POINTS

- Health-related quality of life (HRQoL) is a multidimensional concept based on subjective perception by the patient over the impact of a disease or condition or its treatment on the physical and emotional well-being.
- HRQoL assessment requires the use of validated questionnaires.
- HRQoL is decreased in chronic spontaneous urticaria (especially when associated with angioedema) and in hereditary angioedema caused by C1-inhibitor deficiency (C1-INH-HAE).
- Higher levels in depression and anxiety have been observed in patients with histaminergic angioedema as part of chronic spontaneous urticaria and in patients with C1-INH-HAE compared with general population.
- An important humanistic and economic negative impact has been elucidated in burden of illness studies in C1-INH-HAE, with impairment during angioedema attacks and in free-attacks periods, and affecting patients and caregivers.

Disclosure Statement: T. Caballero has received speaker fees from CSL Behring, GlaxoSmithKline, MSD, Novartis, and Shire; consultancy fees from BioCryst, CSL Behring, Novartis, Shire, and Sobi; funding for travel and meeting attendance from CSL Behring, Novartis, and Shire; and has participated in clinical trials/registries for BioCryst, CSL Behring, Dyax, Novartis, Pharming, and Shire. She is a researcher from the IdiPaz Program for promoting research activities. She is also a coauthor of HAE-QoL and is a researcher from IdiPaz, which owns HAE-QoL copyright. N. Prior has received speaker fees from CSL Behring and Shire; funding for travel and meeting attendance from CSL Behring, Novartis, and Shire; and has participated in clinical trials/registries for CSL Behring, Dyax, and Pharming. She is also coauthor of HAE-QoL questionnaire.

[a] Allergy Department, Hospital La Paz Institute for Health Research (IdiPaz), Paseo de la Castellana 261, Madrid 28046, Spain; [b] CIBERER (U754), Allergy Department, Hospital La Paz Institute for Health Research (IdiPaz), Paseo de la Castellana 261, Madrid 28046, Spain; [c] Allergy Department, Hospital Universitario Severo Ochoa, Avenida de Orellana s/n, Leganés, Madrid 28911, Spain
* Corresponding author. Teresa Caballero, Servicio de Alergia, Hospital Universitario La Paz, Paseo de la Castellana 261, Madrid 28046, Spain.
E-mail address: mteresa.caballero@idipaz.es

Immunol Allergy Clin N Am 37 (2017) 597–616
http://dx.doi.org/10.1016/j.iac.2017.04.005
immunology.theclinics.com

INTRODUCTION

Health-related quality of life (HRQoL) is a term that has been conceptually evolving during the last decades.[1–5] As a simple and summarizing definition one can say that HRQoL is the individual perception of the impact of a disease, disability, or symptom across physical, psychological, social, and somatic domains of functioning and well-being. Evaluating HRQoL is commonly accepted as important for a comprehensive assessment of the patient health status, burden of disease, and treatment response. Its evaluation may help to identify physical, mental, and social health problems not detected in a conventional clinical assessment.[6–8] HRQoL provides essential information in the development of new drugs, health policy planning, and health resources assignment.

The most commonly used tools for measuring HRQoL are questionnaires that comprise several dimensions (physical, social, emotional, cognitive, working, symptoms, treatment secondary effects).[9] HRQoL questionnaires are one type of the denominated patient-reported outcomes, with increasing relevance in patient-centered medicine.[10] HRQoL questionnaires are classified into generic (eg, Short Form 36 Health Survey [SF-36], EuroQol [EQ-5D], Nottingham Health Profile [NHP]) or specific for a certain disease, symptom, or condition.[10,11] Generic questionnaires have the advantage of allowing comparison between different diseases, but usually show a lack of sensitivity when evaluating certain aspects of a particular disease and thus condition-specific questionnaires are usually preferable for this purpose.

When measuring HRQoL it is advisable to use patient-reported outcomes that meet the quality criteria recommended by experts,[12,13] the most important being feasibility, reliability, validity evidences, and sensitivity to change.

HEALTH-RELATED QUALITY-OF-LIFE QUESTIONNAIRES
Generic Questionnaires

Short Form 36 Health Survey
SF-36 is one of the most frequently used generic HRQoL questionnaires. It consists of 36 questions and eight domains (physical functioning, role-physical, bodily pain, general health, vitality, social functioning, role-emotional, and mental health), besides one single item about perceived change in health.[14] The higher the score, the less disability (eg, a score of zero is equivalent to maximum disability and a score of 100 to no disability). One can further examine a summary of physical QoL (physical component summary) and emotional QoL (mental component summary). Subsequently, version 2.0 (SF-36v.2)[15] and two shorter versions (SF-12 and SF-8) have been created.[16,17]

EuroQoL
The EQ-5D consists of three parts: the EQ-5D descriptive system, the EQ visual analog scale, and the EQ-5D index (index value attached to an EQ-5D state according to a particular set of weights).[18] The EQ-5D descriptive system comprises the following five dimensions: mobility, self-care, usual activities, pain/discomfort, and anxiety/depression. Each dimension has three (EQ-5D-3 L) or five severity levels (EQ-5D-5 L). The index-based values (or utilities) are a major feature of the EQ-5D instrument, facilitating the calculation of quality-adjusted life years (QALYs) that are used to inform economic evaluations of health care interventions. There is also a version for children from 7 to 12 years old, called EQ-Youth version (EQ-5D-Y).[19] It is a short and easy tool (it takes 2–3 minutes to be completed) and has been applied in a wide range of health conditions and treatments.

Dermatology-Specific Questionnaires

Among the HRQoL questionnaires for skin disorders one can find tools designed for any skin condition, also called dermatology-specific questionnaires (eg, Dermatology Life Quality Index [DLQI], VQ-Dermato, Skindex-29) and others designed for one specific skin disease (eg, CU-Q_2oL). The characteristics of HRQoL questionnaires used in dermatologic conditions have been revised.[20]

Dermatology Life Quality Index

DLQI is one of the most widely used HRQoL patient-reported outcomes in several dermatologic conditions. It is a 10-item questionnaire that analyzes six subdomains: symptoms and feelings, daily activities, leisure work, school, personal relationships, and treatment. Total score ranges from 0 to 30 (the higher scoring, the higher the HRQoL impairment).[21]

Skindex-29

The Skindex-29 is a 30-item questionnaire with 29 items belonging to three domains (emotions, functioning, symptoms) with separate scores and one remaining item that does not compute to scoring (item 18).[22]

Angioedema-Specific Questionnaires

It is important to consider that generic HRQoL questionnaires are usually not as sensitive as disease-specific ones and thus the use of specific questionnaires is recommended. There are currently two angioedema-specific HRQoL questionnaires available: AE-QoL, specific for angioedema as a symptom[23,24]; and HAE-QoL, specific for adult patients with hereditary angioedema caused by C1-inhibitor deficiency (C1-INH-HAE).[25,26]

AE-QoL

The AE-QoL is a symptom-specific questionnaire developed to assess HRQoL in patients with any kind of recurrent angioedema.[23] It is formed by 17 items grouped into four dimensions: functioning, fatigue/mood, fears/shame, and food[23] and has a recall period of 4 weeks. Patients with different angioedema conditions (chronic spontaneous urticaria [CSU], C1-INH-HAE, idiopathic angioedema) participated in its development. It has shown good psychometric properties with a total internal consistency of 0.89 and a test-retest reliability of 0.83. It comprises a total score and four domain scores ranging from 0 to 100 after a linear transformation of raw scores, with higher scores indicating lower HRQoL.[23]

AE-QoL scores were found to correlate well with DLQI, SF-36, and SF-12 scores,[23,24] and with disease activity.[24] In addition, AE-QoL score changes over time correlated significantly with changes in other AE anchors, thus demonstrating its sensitivity to change. The Minimal Clinically Important Difference (MCID) of the AE-QoL total score was found to be six points.[24] AE-QoL has been applied in some clinical trials in C1-INH-HAE and in CSU.[27,28]

HAE-QoL

The HAE-QoL consists of 25 items and addresses seven relevant HRQoL domains for adult C1-INH-HAE patients (treatment difficulties, physical functioning and health, disease-related stigma, emotional role and social functioning, concern about offspring, perceived control over illness, and mental health).[26] It has been developed following a qualitative methodology, based on a patient-centered perspective. Semi-structured interviews with C1-INH-HAE patients and experts helped to ensure content validity, one of the most important measurement properties. In a first phase the draft version was carried out in a multicenter study in Spain, followed by the internationalization of the questionnaire with 17 participating countries.[25,26] After the international pilot study, the psychometric analysis showed good internal consistency (Cronbach α, 0.92) and test-retest reliability (intraclass correlation coefficient, 0.87), and a good discriminant validity.[26] The assessment for sensitivity to change and MCID is pending.

Other Health-Related Quality-of-Life Measures

Quality-adjusted life-year

The QALY is a measure of the impact of a disease, which includes life length and life quality. It ranges from 1 (year in perfect health status) to 0 (equivalent to death).[29,30] For QALY estimation different elements are considered, the main one being the assignation of preference values for the different health status, also known as utilities. Health status is classified and described to the patient, who assesses and compares them among each other or with death. It is considered that 1 year of life in perfect health condition values 1 (1 year of life × 1 utility value) and half year of life in perfect health status is equal to 0.5 QALY (the same value that 1 year of life in a 0.5 utility value situation [eg, to be confined to bed], 1 year × 0.5 utility value). This measure is frequently used in cost-benefit analysis to calculate the cost ratio per QALY for a certain health intervention, those interventions with a minor ratio being preferable. There are different classification systems for health status, some of them associated with generic instruments, such as the E5QD.[18]

HEALTH-RELATED QUALITY OF LIFE AND BURDEN OF DISEASE IN HISTAMINERGIC ANGIOEDEMA

There are no HRQoL studies in histaminergic angioedema, except those carried out in the context of other conditions, mainly chronic idiopathic urticaria (CIU)/CSU. CSU is defined as the presence of recurrent episodes of wheals (hives) and/or angioedema for at least 6 weeks.[31,32] The proportion of patients with angioedema is variable. Approximately 33% to 67% present hives and angioedema, 29% to 65% only hives, and 1% to 13% angioedema only.[33]

The HRQoL and burden of disease in patients with CSU has been reviewed in different studies.[34–36] HRQoL has been shown to be reduced in patients with CIU/CSU by using generic HRQoL questionnaires (NHP,[37] SF-36[38]), dermatology HRQoL questionnaires (DLQI,[39] Skindex 29[40,41]), and specific HRQoL questionnaires (CU-Q₂oL[42–44]).

Interestingly, a study carried out by O'Donnell and colleagues[37] in the United Kingdom highlighted that 59% of the patients reported that swellings were the worst aspect of their urticaria. Therefore, the presence of angioedema associated to CSU was studied as a possible determinant for higher detriment in HRQoL and the results were contradictory (**Table 1**).

Some studies using DLQI[45,46] and Skindex 29[40] did not find significant differences in HRQoL between patients with only wheals and those with associated angioedema. This could be because DLQI and Skindex 29 are not sensitive enough to detect these differences. However, other studies also using DLQI,[38] or a modified version of DLQI,[47] SF-36,[38] or CU-Q₂oL,[44] found that patients with angioedema had worse QoL than those with only urticaria.

Some studies have shown that patients with CIU/CSU often suffer from depression and anxiety.[48–50] Patients with CIU/CSU and psychiatric comorbidities (anxiety, depression) have significantly reduced HRQoL by using Skindex 29,[40] SF-36,[51] and WHOQOL-BREF.[48,52]

Table 1
Influence of angioedema in HRQoL in patients with CIU/CSU

Authors, Year	Country	HRQoL Instrument	Influence of Angioedema on HRQoL Score
Poon et al,[45] 1999	United Kingdom	DLQI	No influence
Staubach et al,[40] 2006	Germany	Skindex 29	No influence
Ue et al,[38] 2011	Brazil	DLQI SF-36	Worse QoL
Silvares et al,[47] 2011	Brazil	Modified DLQI	Worse QoL
Choi et al,[44] 2016	South Korea	CU-Q2oL	Poorer scores in urticaria domain
Maurer et al,[46] 2016	Germany	DLQI	No influence

HRQoL was assessed by means of DLQI as a secondary efficacy outcome in several clinical trials using omalizumab compared with placebo for CIU/CSU (ASTERIA I, ASTERIA II, GLACIAL). A subanalysis of the patients with angioedema at baseline in these three clinical trials showed that QoL impairment was similar in patients with/without baseline angioedema and that omalizumab, 300 mg, every 4 weeks compared with placebo significantly improved DLQI scores in patients with/without baseline angioedema. This improvement was similar in patients with/without baseline angioedema and was higher than the MCID threshold.[46] QoL improvement by means of CU-Q2oL was the primary objective to evaluate efficacy of omalizumab versus placebo in patients with CSU and angioedema in the X-ACT trial.[53] Omalizumab was superior to placebo in improving CU-Q2oL scores at Week 28 ($P<.001$) and also significantly improved AE-QoL score ($P<.001$).

Regarding economic impact of the disease, Delong and colleagues[54] estimated the annual direct and indirect health care costs in 2008 in the United States. A mean total annual cost of $2047 \pm $1483 was calculated, but it was probably underestimated because over-the-counter medications were not taken into account, or the high costs of treatments in poorly controlled disease. Afterward, another study estimated that the mean whole health care cost was more than $9000 per year.[55]

ASSURE-CSU (Assessment of the Economic and Humanistic Burden of Chronic Spontaneous/Idiopathic Urticaria Patients) is a study that is exploring the economic and humanistic burden in patients diagnosed with CSU/CIU who are symptomatic despite treatment.[56] This study is being performed across seven different countries and is intended to show data on the subgroup of patients with CSU/CIU and angioedema.

HEALTH-RELATED QUALITY OF LIFE AND BURDEN OF DISEASE IN HEREDITARY ANGIOEDEMA CAUSED BY C1-INHIBITOR DEFICIENCY

C1-INH-HAE is the best representative of bradykinin-mediated angioedema.[57] Some characteristics of C1-INH-HAE, such as low prevalence, inheritance, delay in diagnosis, unpredictability of attacks, risk of death caused by asphyxia, pain, unnecessary medical procedures, treatment with ineffective drugs, difficulty in access to specific drugs, and severe side effects with some medications taken as long-term prophylaxis,[58–63] suggest that this disease could significantly decrease HRQoL, but its measurement has only been highlighted in recent years.

The first allusion to HRQoL in C1-INH-HAE in literature is found in 1999, within a study about the HRQoL in several skin conditions with wheals and/or angioedema.[45]

The DLQI was administered to 170 patients, five of them with C1-INH-HAE, and worse HRQoL was observed in C1-INH-HAE patients compared with those with chronic urticaria.

Afterward an online survey performed in the United States to 63 C1-INH-HAE patients[64] identified sudden closure of airway (85%), intolerable pain (65%), and transmission of the disease to children (55%) as the three most frequent major fears of these patients. Besides, level of patient satisfaction on the management of their disease was also explored and 26% of patients considered it was good or satisfactory, whereas 28% only fair and 46% poor or unsatisfactory. It is important to point out that these data were obtained when no specific treatment of C1-INH-HAE was available in the United States.

Several studies used SF-12 or SF-36 to assess HRQoL in patients with C1-INH-HAE. Lumry and colleagues[65] studied HRQoL in US patients with C1-INH-HAE in 2008 and found decreased physical and mental health versus the normative population ($P<.001$) for all subscales and overall physical and mental summary components (**Fig. 1**). At this time no specific treatment of C1-INH-HAE was available in the United States.

Aabom and colleagues[67] used SF-36v2 in 2009 in Denmark and showed that C1-INH-HAE patients rated equally or higher than the normative 1998 US population in all dimensions except in one (general health). Additionally, there was no relationship between C1-INH-HAE severity and SF-36v2 scores.

In Brazil, where danazol was the only financed treatment by the government in 2013, Gomide and colleagues[68] assessed HRQoL by SF-36 in 35 patients. A score less than 70 was observed in 90.4% of the patients, with dimensions of vitality and social role the most affected.

The same year in France, Bouillet and colleagues[69] confirmed the important impairment in HRQoL in C1-INH-HAE patients compared with healthy French population

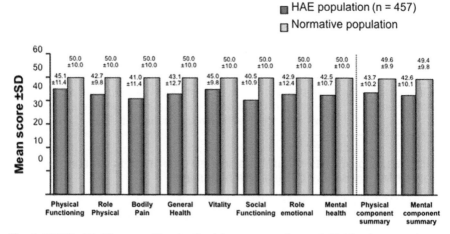

Fig. 1. HRQOL (SF-12) scores. Standardized (*z* score transformed) SF-12 values are shown. Normative population values are based on Ware and colleagues.[66] Patients with HAE reported decreased physical and mental health versus the normative population ($P<.001$) for all subscales and overall summary components, based on *t* tests. SD, standard deviation. (*From* Lumry WR, Castaldo AJ, Vernon MK, et al. The humanistic burden of hereditary angioedema: impact on health-related quality of life, productivity, and depression. Allergy Asthma Proc 2010;31(5):410; with permission.)

(P<.0001) and with allergic patients (P<.05) by also using the SF-36v2. Moreover, they observed that HRQoL negatively correlated with the annual number of attacks and was markedly altered for patients having more than five attacks per year (P<.05).

In 2014, Nordenfelt and colleagues[70] published results from HRQoL in Sweden. Data from children and adult C1-INH-HAE patients were collected by the generic questionnaire EQ5D-5L, for the attack-free state and the last angioedema attack. The patients had a higher score or better HRQoL (mean ± standard deviation, 0.825 ± 0.207) in the attack-free state than during the last attack (mean ± standard deviation, 0.512 ± 0.299; P<.0001). Patients with more than 30 attacks per year had a significantly lower score that those patients with less frequent attacks and it was observed that an increase in the frequency of attacks had also a negative impact on the HRQoL in the periods between attacks. Decreased HRQoL was also detected in women during attack-free periods. In this study results were also compared with those from other chronic diseases characterized by paroxysmal attacks, such as asthma and migraine, with impairment in HRQoL in C1-INH-HAE shown to be higher than in these other two conditions.[70]

Data from C1-INH-HAE impact on HRQoL in 25 family members in Medellin (Colombia) have been recently published.[71] They used the Kidscreen-27 questionnaire in five children (3–17 years old) and the SF-36 questionnaire in 20 adults (23–70 years old). This study showed a higher impact in psychological well-being dimension in children and in the physical role and emotional role dimensions of the SF-36 for adult patients.

Data from studies performed in Denmark, Brazil, and Colombia with SF-36 are shown in **Table 2**. Scores are higher in Denmark, where access to specific drugs is easier. HRQoL results in different countries may be influenced by drug availability and characteristics of health care system. Nevertheless other social and individual factors may be also involved.

In Greece, Psarros and colleagues[72] used a 10-point visual analog scale to assess QoL in patients with C1-INH-HAE and showed that in 14% HAE had influenced their

Table 2
SF-36 scores in different HRQoL studies on C1-INH-HAE

SF-36 Dimension	Denmark (Aabom et al,[67] 2015)	United States 1998 Normative Data (Aabom et al,[67] 2015)	Brazil (Gomide et al,[68] 2013)	Colombia (Sánchez et al,[71] 2015)
Physical functioning	88.7 (±20.8)	83.3 (±23.8)	75.6 (±22.6)	87.1 (±20.4)
Role-physical	85.6 (±23.4)	82.5 (±25.5)	60.6 (±22.0)	17.2 (±11.2)
Bodily pain	78.6 (±24.9)	71.3 (±23.7)	58.1 (±30.1)	67.5 (±31.9)
General health	62.8 (±24.3)	70.8 (±21.0)	59.3 (±18.7)	55.2 (±23.9)
Mental health	81.9 (±14.6)	75.0 (±17.8)	65.72 (±16.8)	51.1 (±28.2)
Role-emotional	89.4 (±24.2)	87.4 (±21.4)	75.9 (±25.1)	11.9 (±10.9)
Social functioning	92.9 (±12.7)	84.3 (±22.9)	54.3 (±13.9)	61.7 (±33.7)
Vitality	66.4 (±21.8)	58.3 (±20.0)	51.0 (±12.4)	54.5 (±21.1)
PCS	NA	NA	NA	49.2 (±9.5)
MCS	NA	NA	NA	29.1 (±11.9)

Abbreviations: MCS, mental component summary; NA, not available; PCS, physical component summary.

QoL slightly (0–3), in 63% greatly (4–7), and in 23% significantly (8–10). They also used a specific questionnaire to find out which disease-specific factors were reported by the patients to affect their QoL.

In the last years, interest in the impact of C1-INH-HAE on HRQoL in the context of therapeutic interventions or the development of new drugs has increased. Bygum and colleagues[73] applied SF-36v2 and DLQI to evaluate the effect of home self-administration of intravenous plasma-derived C1-inhibitor concentrate (pdhC1INH) in HRQoL. The authors compared the SF-36 and DLQI scores before and after home therapy and observed an improvement in HRQoL after intervention on physical and psychological parameters.[73] The mean DLQI score fell from 12.6 ± 4.65 to 2.7 ± 1.38 (P<.001), whereas the mean SF-36 scores for the individual domains also improved significantly, and for physical component summary and mental component summary (30.95–51.96 and 39.08–58.99, respectively).[73]

Likewise, Kreuz and colleagues[74] also demonstrated improvement in HRQoL after pdhC1INH self-administration by using an adaptation of the Pain Disability Index in 22 patients with severe angioedema attacks without good control under maintenance treatment with danazol. Danazol treatment was replaced with home self-administered C1INH concentrate and all the HRQoL-related variables addressed by the questionnaire improved significantly.

Several years later, Aabom and colleagues[67] applied SF-36v2 to compare HRQoL in patients under pdhC1INH self-administration program versus non-self-injecting patients. They did not find statistically significant differences, except for the General Health dimension that showed a significant lower score in the self-injecting group. The authors considered these findings mainly caused by two factors: home treatment could act as a frequent reminder of the chronic disease despite having many benefits; and self-injecting is commonly offered to patients with more severe clinical expression of the disease.

Moreover, Squeglia and colleagues[75] compared HRQoL by means of HAE-QoL in patients receiving home self-treatment with pdhC1INH or icatibant versus patients receiving hospital treatment with pdhC1INH, and surprisingly found that C1-INH-HAE patients receiving treatment at hospital had higher HRQoL. Larger studies should be done and possible confounding factors, such as attack frequency, should be analyzed.

In the context of the clinical trial I.M.P.A.C.T. 2 by CSL-Behring (Marburg, Germany) in the United States, Bewtra and colleagues[76] assessed HRQoL with SF-12. Eighteen subjects gave their feedback about their HRQoL while being treated with pdhC1INH. Mean scores ranged from 44.5 to 93.4 with only one subject having an SF-12 score of less than 50. One of the limitations of this study is that there was no control group and no data were collected to compare HRQoL before and after the availability of pdhC1INH.

SF-36 survey (version 1.0) was used in a multicenter, randomized, placebo-controlled, crossover clinical trial (NCT01005888) in which 22 patients received either intravenous injections of 1000 U of pdhC1INH (Cinryze, Shire HGT, Zug, Switzerland) or placebo every 3 to 4 days for 12 weeks and then crossed over to the other treatment arm for a second 12-week period. These patients could also be treated open-label with C1 INH-nf (Cinryze; 1000 U) for the acute treatment of angioedema attacks in both arms of the study. SF-36 was administered at the beginning and end of the two 12-week treatment periods and 16 patients had evaluable SF-36 data. A significant increase in both physical and mental component summaries was found after active treatment period with respect to baseline and placebo.[77]

In a randomized clinical trial with avoralstat (BioCryst Pharmaceuticals, Durham, NC), an oral kallikrein inhibitor, C1-INH-HAE patients showed an improvement in the four dimensions of the AE-QoL compared with nearly no improvement during placebo treatment.[26]

Bygum[78] analyzed the impact of C1-INH-HAE before and after creating a comprehensive HAE center in Denmark. More than half of the patients reported that the disease had a significant psychological impact on their lives and restricted their physical activities. Home treatment with pdhC1INH reduced the illness burden.

The first comprehensive burden of illness study in C1-INH-HAE was carried out in the United States in 2007 to 2008 with the collaboration of the United States Hereditary Angioedema Association and financed by Dyax corporation (currently part of Shire HGT, Zug, Switzerland[65]; HAE-BoI-USA study). C1-INH-HAE burden was assessed via a World Wide Web–based survey completed by 457 patients. C1-INH-HAE patients reported decreased HRQoL as described previously.

This study also revealed reduced productivity and missed opportunities because of C1-INH-HAE. Approximately half of the patients (50.6%) working full or part-time had missed at least 1 day of work because of their most recent angioedema attack and 44.4% of students had missed at least 1 school day.[65] Workers had missed a mean of 3.3 days of work and students a mean of 1.9 days of school because of their most recent angioedema attack. Reduced productivity determined by the Work Productivity and Activity in Impairment-General Health questionnaire in C1-INH-HAE patients was comparable with that experienced by patients with severe asthma or Crohn's disease (**Fig. 2**). Furthermore, 59.33% of participants reported that they had missed at least 1 day of leisure activities as a result of their most recent angioedema attack.

The HAE-BoI-USA study also assessed the direct and indirect economic costs associated with acute attacks and long-term management of C1-INH-HAE.[79] Total annual per-patient costs were estimated at $42,000 for the average C1-INH-HAE patient. Direct costs came to approximately to $26,000 annually, the largest component

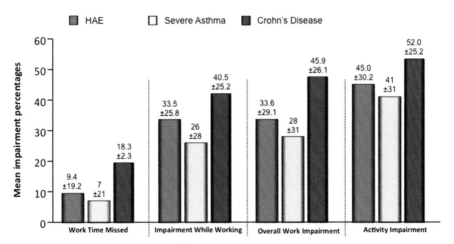

Fig. 2. Impact of C1-INH-HAE on productivity. Mean impairment percentages (±standard deviation) as determined by the Work Productivity and Activity in Impairment-General Health are presented. The reduced productivity experienced by patients with HAE is comparable with that experienced by patients with severe asthma or Crohn's disease, as reported in the literature. (*From* Lumry WR, Castaldo AJ, Vernon MK, et al. The humanistic burden of hereditary angioedema: impact on health-related quality of life, productivity, and depression. Allergy Asthma Proc 2010;31(5):411; with permission.)

because of hospital stays for acute attacks (67%). Respondents reported high rates of missed work, lost productivity, and lost income, contributing to indirect costs totaling $16,000 annually for the average patient.

Afterward, a burden of illness study was carried out in Europe in 2011 (HAE-Bol-Europe study), with participation of 186 patients from Denmark, Germany, and Spain.[80–84] The study was funded by Viropharma SPRL (currently part of Shire HGT, Zug, Switzerland).

Patients were recruited from HAE centers of excellence and from HAE patient associations in each country. It was shown that C1-INH-HAE had a high impact over patients' daily activities and over patients and caregivers' productivity during attacks. A decrease in productivity was also observed between attacks, which was greater with a higher frequency of angioedema attacks. The school/work absenteeism caused by the last angioedema attack is shown in **Fig. 3**.

In addition, in the HAE-Bol-USA study[65] and in the HAE-Bol-Europe study[82] a significant percentage of the participants revealed that C1-INH-HAE had hindered their career and/or educational advancement, and prevented them from applying to certain jobs (**Fig. 4**).

In the HAE-Bol-Europe study, open-ended patient interviews were carried out with 30 C1-INH-HAE patients.[83] Qualitative analysis of data yielded five main areas that characterize the burden in this disease: unnecessary treatments and procedures, symptom triggers, attack impacts, caregiver impacts, and long-term impacts. Based on these findings a conceptual model was developed, illustrating the hypothesized relationships among the wide-ranging short- and long-term HRQoL impacts of C1-INH-HAE and that may be useful to highlight important issues in clinical management

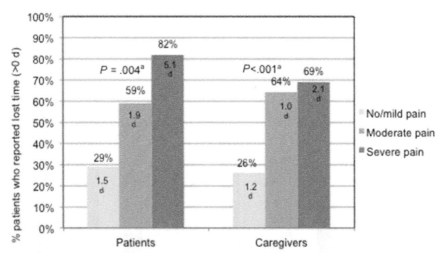

Fig. 3. Work/school absenteeism during last attack by pain severity. Percentage who missed time and reported mean days missed. [a] P values for difference in percentage that missed time. Percentages based on 72 patients who were employed or in school and provided absenteeism data. Percent of caregivers based on full sample (N = 164). Means based on number of patients (n = 40) and caregivers (n = 86) who missed time. Caregiver time includes leisure time. Data missing for missed time for 31 caregivers. (*From* Aygören-Pürsün E, Bygum A, Beusterien K, et al. Socioeconomic burden of hereditary angioedema: results from the hereditary angioedema burden of illness study in Europe. Orphanet J Rare Dis 2014;99; with permission.)

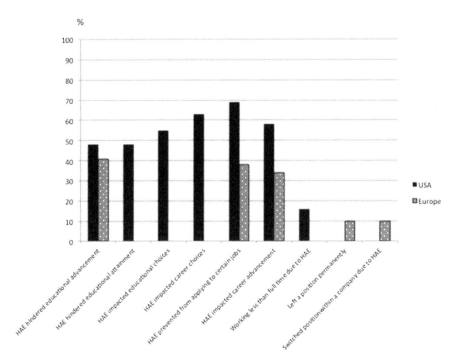

Fig. 4. Missed opportunities because of C1-INH-HAE. Combined data from the HAE-Bol-USA study[65] and the HAE-Bol-Europe study.[82] (*Data from* Lumry WR, Castaldo AJ, Vernon MK, et al. The humanistic burden of hereditary angioedema: impact on health-related quality of life, productivity, and depression. Allergy Asthma Proc 2010;31(5):407–14; and Aygören-Pürsün E, Bygum A, Beusterien K, et al. Socioeconomic burden of hereditary angioedema: results from the hereditary angioedema burden of illness study in Europe. Orphanet J Rare Dis 2014;9:99.)

(Fig. 5).[83] Banerji[84] and Bonner and colleagues[85] proposed other conceptual models for C1-INH-HAE.

Aygören-Pürsün and colleagues[86] estimated health status utilities (preference) weights in the HAE-Bol-Europe study in patients with C1-INH-HAE from Denmark, Germany, and Spain. They manually cross-walked some survey items to the EQ-5D domains (pain/discomfort, mobility, self-care, usual activities, and anxiety/depression) and compared them with the UK population-based EQ-5D utility weights. The mean utilities for the last AE attack were 0.44 and increased to 0.72 between attacks. Besides, utilities for the last attack depended on the severity of pain of that attack (0.61 for no pain or mild pain, 0.47 for moderate pain, and 0.08 for severe pain). There were no significant differences across countries. The authors concluded that C1-INH-HAE produces meaningful health status disabilities associated with acute attacks and between attacks from the patient perspective.

Furthermore, some studies analyzed different individual aspects of the economic burden of C1-INH-HAE.[87,88]

Different studies have described higher levels of depression and/or anxiety in C1-INH-HAE patients compared with the general population. Lumry and colleagues[65] observed in the HAE-Bol-USA study that C1-INH-HAE patients had higher depression scores than population norms by using the Hamilton Depression Inventory-Short Form

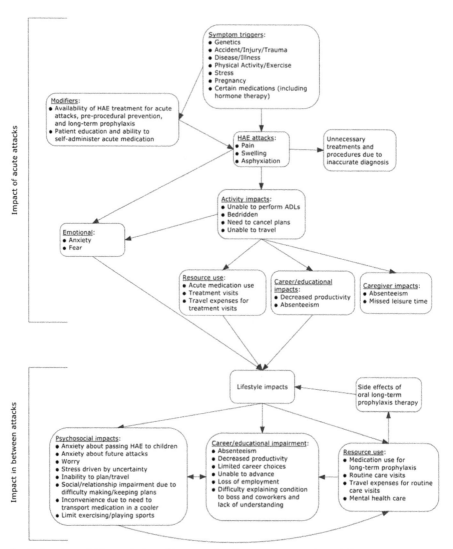

Fig. 5. Burden of illness in hereditary angioedema: conceptual model. ADL, activities of daily living. (*From* Bygum A, Aygören-Pürsün E, Beusterien K, et al. Burden of illness in hereditary angioedema: a conceptual model. Acta Derm Venereol 2015;95(6):708; with permission.)

(8.1 ± 6.5 vs 3.1 ± 3.0; *P*<.001), with 42.5% of the patients scoring greater than 8.5, indicative of depressive symptomatology. Afterward, a study about prevalence of depression and anxiety in C1-INH-HAE patients was also carried out in the United States by using the Hamilton Depression Rating Scale and the Hamilton Anxiety Scale.[89] In this study 39% of the respondents showed clinically significant depressive symptoms (19.23% mild, 15.38% moderate, and 3.85% severe). Fifteen percent of participants displayed prominent anxiety (50% mild, 25% moderate, and 25% severe). Finally, a total of 19.5% of the participant patients in the HAE-Bol-USA study were

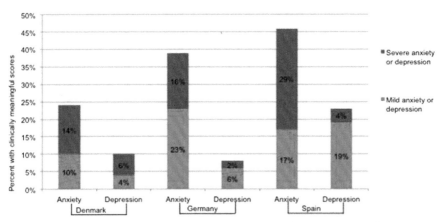

Fig. 6. Hospital Anxiety and Depression Scale scores. Possible scores range from 0 to 21. Scores of ≤7 indicate the absence of anxiety/depression. Scores of 8–10 indicate mild anxiety/depression and scores of ≥11 indicate moderate-to-severe anxiety/depression. (*From* Caballero T, Aygören-Pürsün E, Bygum A, et al. The humanistic burden of hereditary angioedema: results from the burden of illness study in Europe. Allergy Asthma Proc 2014;35(1):5; with permission.)

under treatment with psychotropic or antidepressant medication, which was nearly double the national average of 11.1%.[65]

In the HAE-BoI-Europe study the levels of depression and anxiety were also assessed by means of the Hospital Anxiety and Depression Scales.[81] Thirty-eight

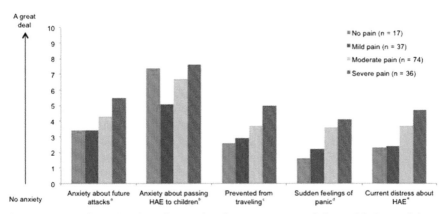

Fig. 7. HAE-specific anxiety by pain severity of most recent attack (n = 164). For each item, differences in anxiety among pain severity levels are statistically significant ($P<.05$ for each item). [a] How anxious are you about having an attack in the future? [b] How anxious are you about the potential of transferring HAE to your children? [c] How much does HAE prevent you from going on vacation/traveling? [d] How often did you get sudden feelings of panic about HAE symptoms/attacks during the past 6 months?; rescaled from a 5-point Likert scale to a 0–10 scale. [e] How distressed are you about your HAE attacks/symptoms?; rescaled from a five-point Likert scale to a 0–10 scale. (*From* Caballero T, Aygören-Pürsün E, Bygum A, et al. The humanistic burden of hereditary angioedema: results from the burden of illness study in Europe. Allergy Asthma Proc 2014;35(1):5; with permission.)

Table 3
HRQoL patient-reported outcomes used in C1-INH-HAE

	General Tools			Dermatologic Tools	AE Tools	HAE Tools	Other Tools
	SF-12	SF-36v2	ESQD	DLQI	AE-QoL	HAE-QoL[a]	Pain Disability Index[c]
Recall period	1 mo (1 wk)	4 wk (1 wk)	1 d	1 wk	4 wk	6 mo	Not specified
No. items	12	36	5/1	10	17	25	7
Completion time	10–15 min	10–15 min		126 sg	<5 min	[a]	
Validated for HAE	No	No	No	No	[b]	Yes	No
Score	0–100	0–100		0–30	0–100	25–135	0–60[c]
Age				≥16	≥18	≥18	≥18
Dimensions	8	8	6	6	4	7	6[c]
	• Physical function • Role physical • Bodily pain • General health • Mental health • Role emotional • Social functions • Vitality	• Physical function • Role physical • Bodily pain • General health • Mental health • Role emotional • Social functions • Vitality	• Family/home responsibility • Social activities • Occupation • Life support activity • General condition • Condition during attacks	• Symptoms and feelings • Daily activities • Leisure • Work and school • Personal relationships • Treatment	• Functioning • Fatigue/mood • Fears/shame • Food	• Physical functioning and health • Role emotional and social functioning • Concern about offspring • Treatment difficulties • Disease-related stigma • Perceived control over illness • Mental health	• Family/home responsibility • Social activities • Occupation • Life support activity • General condition • Condition during attacks

a 44-item HAE-QoL version: mean ± standard deviation, 26.0 ± 2.7 min; median, 19 min (range, 5–180 min; interquartile range, 12.5–30.0).
b Validated for angioedema as a symptom and not for C1-INH-HAE: (1) open interviews, 3 of 10 patients with C1-INH-HAE; (2) item reduction, 21 of 110 patients with C1-INH-HAE.
c An adaptation of the Pain Disability Index was used.[74] Six instead of seven domains were applied and the score ranged from 0 to 60 instead of 0 to 70.

percent and 14% of the patients had clinically meaningful anxiety and depression, respectively. Anxiety levels were higher compared with general population, but not depression levels. Anxiety and depression scores were higher in Spain than in the other two countries (**Fig. 6**).

In this study anxiety regarding five specific C1-INH-HAE items was explored. Anxiety associated with each item was directly correlated with the pain severity of their most recent attack ($P<0.05$), except anxiety regarding passing the disease to their children, which was rated high even among patients who reported no pain during their last attack (**Fig. 7**).

The regression model showed that attack severity, frequency, duration of swelling, and country of residence were significant predictors of higher anxiety related to C1-INH-HAE. Spanish and German patients had worse HAE-specific anxiety scores than Danish patients ($P<.02$).

Banerji and colleagues[90] performed in 2013 a survey in collaboration with the United States Hereditary Angioedema Association to improve the understanding of the state of HAE care from the patient perspective after the introduction of new specific treatments for C1-INH-HAE. In this study 72% of patients with C1-INH-HAE reported that HAE produced a significant impact on their QoL despite improved access to effective treatments.

Christiansen and colleagues[91] intended to study if the availability of effective treatment of acute attacks was able to transform the care of HAE patients. Patients were asked to rate the burden of HAE at that moment and compare by recall with 2009 when these therapies were not available in the United States. Specific questions of the survey included five domains: psychological/emotional status, ability to carry out daily activities, fear of suffocation, worry about their children inheriting HAE, and medication side effects. Burden of disease showed significant improvement in all domains except worry about children inheriting HAE. The improvement was higher in those patients with more severe burden of illness, but burden of illness remained.

In summary, C1-INH-HAE is associated with a significant and multifaceted disease burden.[65,83,85] C1-INH-HAE experts recommend that HRQoL be measured on an annual basis[92] and World Allergy Organization C1-INH-HAE guidelines state that HRQoL should be considered when assessing the need for maintenance treatment.[93] A summary of the HRQoL instruments used in C1-INH-HAE is shown in **Table 3**.

HEALTH-RELATED QUALITY OF LIFE AND BURDEN OF DISEASE IN OTHER BRADYKININ-INDUCED ANGIOEDEMAS

There is only one published reference to burden of disease in nC1-INH-HAE.[90] In this study 76% of the patients with nC1-INH-HAE reported that the disease had a significant impact on their QoL, similar to the 72% in C1-INH-HAE.

To our knowledge, there have been no studies on burden of disease and HRQoL in other types of bradykinergic angioedema, such as acquired angioedema caused by C1-INH deficiency and angioedema related to angiotensin converting enzyme inhibitors.

FUTURE CONSIDERATIONS/SUMMARY

Histaminergic angioedema in the context of CSU and C1-INH-HAE have a negative impact on patient HRQoL and produce a significant humanistic and economic burden. Additional burden of illness studies are necessary to assess the impact of different types of angioedema on HRQoL and determine if new interventions and treatments improve this parameter.

REFERENCES

1. Preamble to the Constitution of the World Health Organization as adopted by the International Health Conference, New York, 19-22 June, 1946; signed on 22 July 1946 by the representatives of 61 States (Official Records of the World Health Organization, no. 2, p. 100) and entered into force on 7 April 1948.
2. Kaplan R, Bush J. Health-related quality of life measurement for evaluation research and policy analysis. Health Psychol 1982;1:61–80.
3. Patrick D, Erickson P. What constitutes quality of life? Concepts and dimensions. Qual Life Cardiovasc Care 1988;4:103–26.
4. Schipper H, Clinch J, Powell V. Definition and conceptual issues. In: Spilker B, editor. Quality of life assessments in clinical trials, vol. 4. New York: Raven Press; 1990. p. 11–25.
5. Revicki D, Osoba D, Faiclough D, et al. Recommendations on health-related quality of life research to support labeling and promotional claims in United States. Qual Life Res 2000;9:887–900.
6. Detmar S, Muller M, Schornagel J, et al. Health-related quality of life assessments and patient-physician communication: a randomised controlled trial. JAMA 2002; 288:3027–34.
7. Fung C, Hays R. Prospects and challenges in using patient-reported outcomes in clinical practice. Qual Life Res 2008;17:1297–302.
8. Higginson I, Carr A. Measuring quality of life: using quality of life measures in the clinical setting. BMJ 2001;313(7297):1297–300.
9. Testa M, Simonson D. Assessment of quality-of-life outcomes. N Engl J Med 1996;334:835–40.
10. U. S. Department of Health and Human Services, Food and Drug Administration. Center for Drug Evaluation and Research (CDER), Center for Biologics Evaluation and Research (CBER), Center for Devices and Radiological Health (CDRH). Guidance for industry. Patient-reported outcome measures: use in medical product development to support labeling claims; 2009. Available at: http://www.fda.gov/downloads/Drugs/Guidances/UCM193282.pdfhttp://www.fda.gov/downloads/Drugs/Guidances/UCM193282.pdf Accessed December 12, 2016.
11. Patrick D, Deyo R. Generic and disease-specific measures in assessing health status and quality of life. Med Care 1989;27:S217–32.
12. Reeve BB, Wyrwich KW, Wu AW, et al. ISOQOL recommends minimum standards for patient-reported outcome measures used in patient-centered outcomes and comparative effectiveness research. Qual Life Res 2013;22:1889–905.
13. Mokkink LB, Terwee CB, Patrick DL, et al. The COSMIN checklist for assessing the methodological quality of studies on measurement properties of health status measurement instruments: an international Delphi study. Qual Life Res 2010;19: 539–49.
14. Ware E, Sherbourne CD. The MOS 36 item short-form health survey (SF-36). Conceptual framework and item selection. Med Care 1992;30:473–83.
15. Ware JJ, Kosinski M, Bjorner J, et al. User's manual for the SF-36v2TM health survey. 2nd edition. Lincoln (RI): Quality Metric Incorporated; 2007.
16. Ware J Jr, Kosinski M, Keller SD. A 12-Item Short-Form Health Survey: construction of scales and preliminary tests of reliability and validity. Med Care 1996;34: 220–33.
17. Ware JE Jr, Kosinski M, Dewey JE, et al. How to score and interpret single-item health status measures: a manual for users of the SF-8TM Health Survey. Lincoln (RI): Quality Metric Incorporated; 2001.

18. EuroQoL Group. EuroQol: a new facility for the measurement of health-related quality of life. Health Policy 1990;16:199–208.
19. EuroQoL group. EQ-5D products. Available at: http://www.euroqol.org/eq-5d-products.html. Accessed December 12, 2016.
20. Both H, Essink-Bot ML, Busschbach J, et al. Critical review of generic and dermatology-specific health-related quality of life instruments. J Invest Dermatol 2007;127:2726–39.
21. Finlay A, Khan G. Dermatology life quality index (DLQI): a simple practical measure for routine clinical use. Clin Exp Dermatol 1994;19:210–6.
22. Chren MM, Lasek RJ, Flocke SA, et al. Improved discriminative and evaluative capability of a refined version of Skindex, a quality-of-life instrument for patients with skin diseases. Arch Dermatol 1997;133:1433–40.
23. Weller K, Groffik A, Magerl M, et al. Development and construct validation of the angioedema quality of life questionnaire. Allergy 2012;67:1289–98.
24. Weller K, Magerl M, Peveling-Oberhag A, et al. The angioedema quality of life questionnaire (AE-QoL): assessment of sensitivity to change and minimal clinically important difference. Allergy 2016;71:1203–9.
25. Prior N, Remor E, Gómez-Traseira C, et al. Development of a disease-specific quality of life questionnaire for adult patients with hereditary angioedema due to C1 inhibitor deficiency (HAE-QoL): Spanish multi-centre research project. Health Qual Life Outcomes 2012;10:82.
26. Prior N, Remor E, Pérez-Fernández E, et al. Psychometric field study of hereditary angioedema quality of life questionnaire for adults: HAE-QoL. J Allergy Clin Immunol Pract 2016;4:464–73.e4.
27. Aygören-Pürsün E, Magerl M, Graff J, et al. Prophylaxis of hereditary angioedema attacks: a randomized trial of oral plasma kallikrein inhibition with avoralstat. J Allergy Clin Immunol 2016;138:934–6.e5.
28. Koch K, Weller K, Werner A, et al. Antihistamine updosing reduces disease activity in difficult-to-treat cholinergic urticaria. J Allergy Clin Immunol 2016;138:1483–5.e9.
29. Mehrez A, Gafni A. Quality-adjusted life years, utility theory, and healthy-years equivalents. Med Decis Making 1989;9:142–9.
30. Smith M, Drummond M, Brixner D. Moving the QALY forward: rationale for change. Value Health 2009;12(Suppl 1):S1–4.
31. Bernstein JA, Lang DM, Khan DA, et al. The diagnosis and management of acute and chronic urticaria: 2014 update. J Allergy Clin Immunol 2014;133:1270–7.
32. Zuberbier T, Aberer W, Asero R, et al. The EAACI/GA(2) LEN/EDF/WAO Guideline for the definition, classification, diagnosis, and management of urticaria: the 2013 revision and update. Allergy 2014;69:868–87.
33. Maurer M, Weller K, Bindslev-Jensen C, et al. Unmet clinical needs in chronic spontaneous urticaria. A GA2LEN task force report. Allergy 2011;66:317–30.
34. Weldon D. Quality of life in patients with urticaria and angioedema: assessing burden of disease. Allergy Asthma Proc 2014;35:4–9.
35. O'Donnell BF. Urticaria: impact on quality of life and economic cost. Immunol Allergy Clin North Am 2014;34:89–104.
36. Weller K, Siebenhaar F, Hawro T, et al. Clinical measures of chronic urticaria. Immunol Allergy Clin North Am 2017;37:35–49.
37. O'Donnell BF, Lawlor F, Simpsom J, et al. The impact of chronic urticaria on the quality of life. Br J Dermatol 1997;136:197–201.
38. Ue AP, Souza PK, Rotta O, et al. Quality of life assessment in patients with chronic urticaria. An Bras Dermatol 2011;86:897–904.

39. Basra MK, Fenech R, Gatt RM, et al. The dermatology life quality index 1994-2007: a comprehensive review of validation data and clinical results. Br J Dermatol 2008;159:997–1035.

40. Staubach P, Eckhardt-Henn A, Dechene M, et al. Quality of life in patients with chronic urticaria is differentially impaired and determined by psychiatric comorbidity. Br J Dermatol 2006;154:294–8.

41. Maurer M, Ortonne JP, Zuberbier T. Chronic urticaria: a patient survey on quality-of-life, treatment usage and doctor-patient relation. Allergy 2009;64:581–8.

42. Baiardini I, Pasquali M, Braido F, et al. A new tool to evaluate the impact of chronic urticaria on quality of life: chronic urticaria quality of life questionnaire (CU-QoL). Allergy 2005;60:1073–8.

43. Młynek A, Magerl M, Hanna M, et al. The German version of the chronic urticaria quality-of-life questionnaire: factor analysis, validation, and initial clinical findings. Allergy 2009;64:927–36.

44. Choi WS, Lim ES, Ban GY, et al. Disease-specific impairment of the quality of life in adult patients with chronic spontaneous urticaria. Korean J Intern Med 2016. http://dx.doi.org/10.3904/kjim.2015.195.

45. Poon E, Seed P, Greaves M, et al. The extent and nature of disability in different urticarial conditions. Br J Dermatol 1999;140:667–71.

46. Maurer M, Sofen H, Ortiz B, et al. Positive impact of omalizumab on angioedema and quality of life in patients with refractory chronic idiopathic/spontaneous urticaria: analyses according to the presence or absence of angioedema. J Eur Acad Dermatol Venereol 2016. http://dx.doi.org/10.1111/jdv.14075.

47. Silvares MR, Fortes MR, Miot HA. Quality of life in chronic urticaria: a survey at a public university outpatient clinic, Botucatu (Brazil). Rev Assoc Med Bras (1992) 2011;57:577–82 [in English, Portuguese].

48. Engin B, Uguz F, Yilmaz E, et al. The levels of depression, anxiety and quality of life in patients with chronic idiopathic urticaria. J Eur Acad Dermatol Venereol 2008;22:36–40.

49. Uguz F, Engin B, Yilmaz E. Quality of life in patients with chronic idiopathic urticaria: the impact of axis I and axis II psychiatric disorders. Gen Hosp Psychiatry 2008;30:453–7.

50. Staubach P, Dechene M, Metz M, et al. High prevalence of mental disorders and emotional distress in patients with chronic spontaneous urticaria. Acta Derm Venereol 2011;91:557–61.

51. Ozkan M, Oflaz SB, Kocaman N, et al. Psychiatric morbidity and quality of life in patients with chronic idiopathic urticaria. Ann Allergy Asthma Immunol 2007;99:29–33.

52. Uguz F, Engin B, Yilmaz E, et al. II diagnoses in patients with chronic idiopathic urticaria. J Psychosom Res 2008;64:225–9.

53. Staubach P, Metz M, Chapman-Rothe N, et al. Effect of omalizumab on angioedema in H1-antihistamine-resistant chronic spontaneous urticaria patients: results from X-ACT, a randomized controlled trial. Allergy 2016;71:1135–44.

54. Delong LK, Culler SD, Saini SS, et al. Annual direct and indirect health care costs of chronic idiopathic urticaria: a cost analysis of 50 nonimmunosuppressed patients. Arch Dermatol 2008;144:35–9.

55. Broder MS, Raimundo K, Antonova E, et al. Resource use and costs in an insured population of patients with chronic idiopathic/spontaneous urticaria. Am J Clin Dermatol 2015;16:313–21.

56. Weller K, Maurer M, Grattan C, et al. ASSURE-CSU: a real-world study of burden of disease in patients with symptomatic chronic spontaneous urticaria. Clin Transl Allergy 2015;5:29.

57. Cicardi M, Aberer W, Banerji A, et al. Classification, diagnosis, and approach to treatment for angioedema: consensus report from the Hereditary Angioedema International Working Group. Allergy 2014;69:602–16.

58. Agostoni A, Cicardi M. Hereditary and acquired C1-inhibitor deficiency: biological and clinical characteristics in 235 patients. Medicine 1992;71:206–15.

59. Cicardi M, Castelli R, Zingale L, et al. Side effects of long-term prophylaxis with attenuated androgens in hereditary angioedema: comparison of treated and untreated patients. J Allergy Clin Immunol 1997;99:194–6.

60. Bork K, Pitton M, Harten P, et al. Hepatocellular adenomas in patients taking danazol for hereditary angio-oedema. Lancet 1999;353:1066–7.

61. Bork K, Meg G, Staubach P, et al. Hereditary angioedema: new findings concerning symptoms, affected organs and course. Am J Med 2006;119:267–74.

62. Zuraw B. Hereditary angioedema. N Engl J Med 2008;359:1027–36.

63. Bork K, Hardt J, Witzke G. Fatal laryngeal attacks and mortality in hereditary angioedema due to C1-inhibitor deficiency. J Allergy Clin Immunol 2012;130:692–7.

64. Huang S. Results of an on-line survey of patients with hereditary angioedema. Allergy Asthma Proc 2004;25:127–31.

65. Lumry W, Castaldo A, Vernon M, et al. The humanistic burden of hereditary angioedema: impact on health-related quality of life, productivity, and depression. Allergy Asthma Proc 2010;31:407–14.

66. Ware JE Jr, Kosinski M, Turner-Bowker D, et al. How to score version 2 of the SF-12 health survey (with a supplement documenting version 1). Lincoln (RI): Quality Metric, Inc; 2002.

67. Aabom A, Andersen KE, Perez-Fernández E, et al. Health-related quality of life in Danish patients with hereditary angioedema. Acta Derm Venereol 2015;95:225–6.

68. Gomide M, Toledo E, Valle S, et al. Hereditary angioedema: quality of life in Brazilian patients. Clinics (Sao Paulo) 2013;68:81–3.

69. Bouillet L, Launay D, Fain O, et al. Hereditary angioedema with C1 inhibitor deficiency: clinical presentation and quality of life of 193 French patients. Ann Allergy Asthma Immunol 2013;111:290–4.

70. Nordenfelt P, Dawson S, Wahlgren C-F, et al. Quantifying the burden of disease and perceived health state in patients with hereditary angioedema in Sweden. Allergy Asthma Proc 2014;35:185–90.

71. Sánchez M, Cuervo J, Rave D, et al. Angioedema hereditario en medellin, (Colombia): evaluación clínica y de la calidad de vida. Biomedica 2015;35: 419–28.

72. Psarros F, Koutsostathis N, Farmaki E, et al. Hereditary angioedema in Greece: the first results of the Greek hereditary angioedema registry. Int Arch Allergy Immunol 2014;164:326–32.

73. Bygum A, Andersen K, Mikkelsen C. Self-administration of intravenous C1-inhibitor therapy for hereditary angioedema and associated quality of life benefits. Eur J Dermatol 2009;19:147–51.

74. Kreuz W, Martínez-Saguer I, Aygören-Pürsün E, et al. C1-inhibitor concentrate for individual replacement therapy in patients with severe hereditary angioedema refractory to danazol prophylaxis. Transfusion 2009;49:1987–95.

75. Squeglia V, Barbarino A, Bova M, et al. High attack frequency in patients with angioedema due to C1-inhibitor deficiency is a major determinant in switching to home therapy: a real-life observational study. Orphanet J Rare Dis 2016;11:133.

76. Bewtra A, Levy R, Jacobson K, et al. C1-inhibitor therapy for hereditary angioedema attacks: prospective assessments of health-related quality of life. Allergy Asthma Proc 2012;33:427–31.

77. Lumry WR, Miller DP, Newcomer S, et al. Quality of life in patients with hereditary angioedema receiving therapy for routine prevention of attacks. Allergy Asthma Proc 2014;35:371–6.

78. Bygum A. Hereditary angioedema: consequences of a new treatment paradigm in Denmark. Acta Derm Venereol 2014;94:436–41.

79. Wilson DA, Bork K, Shea EP, et al. Economic costs associated with acute attacks and long-term management of hereditary angioedema. Ann Allergy Asthma Immunol 2010;104:314–20.

80. Bygum A, Aygören-Pürsün E, Beusterien K, et al. The hereditary angioedema Burden Of illness Study in Europe (HAE BOIS-Europe): background and methodology. BMC Dermatol 2012;12:4.

81. Caballero T, Aygören-Pürsün E, Bygum A, et al. The humanistic burden of hereditary angioedema: results from burden of illness study in Europe. Allergy Asthma Proc 2014;35:47–53.

82. Aygören-Pürsün E, Bygum A, Beusterien K, et al. Socioeconomic burden of hereditary angioedema: results from the hereditary angioedema burden of illness study in Europe. Orphanet J Rare Dis 2014;9:99.

83. Bygum A, Aygören-Pürsün E, Beusterien K, et al. Burden of illness in hereditary angioedema: a conceptual model. Acta Derm Venereol 2015;95:706–10.

84. Banerji A. The burden of illness in patients with hereditary angioedema. Ann Allergy Asthma Immunol 2013;111:329–36.

85. Bonner N, Abetz-Webb L, Renault L, et al. Development and content validity testing of a patient-reported outcomes questionnaire for the assessment of hereditary angioedema in observational studies. Health Qual Life Outcomes 2015;13:92.

86. Aygören-Pürsün E, Bygum A, Beusterien K, et al. Estimation of EuroQol 5-Dimensions health status utility values in hereditary angioedema. Patient Prefer Adherence 2016;10:1699–707.

87. Blasco AJ, Lázaro P, Caballero T, et al. Social costs of icatibant self-administration vs. health professional-administration in the treatment of hereditary angioedema in Spain. Health Econ Rev 2013;3:2.

88. Kawalec P, Holko P, Paszulewicz A. Cost-utility analysis of Ruconest (conestat alfa) compared to Berinert P (human C1 esterase inhibitor) in the treatment of acute, life-threatening angioedema attacks in patients with hereditary angioedema. Postepy Dermatol Alergol 2013;30:152–8.

89. Fouche AS, Saunders EFH, Craig T. Depression and anxiety in patients with hereditary angioedema. Ann Allergy Asthma Immunol 2014;112(4):371–5.

90. Banerji A, Busse P, Christiansen SC, et al. Current state of hereditary angioedema management: a patient survey. Allergy Asthma Proc 2015;36:213–7.

91. Christiansen SC, Bygum A, Banerji A, et al. Before and after, the impact of available on-demand treatment for HAE. Allergy Asthma Proc 2015;36:145–50.

92. Cicardi M, Bork K, Caballero T, et al. Evidence-based recommendations for the therapeutic management of angioedema owing to hereditary C1 inhibitor deficiency: consensus report of an International Working Group. Allergy 2012;67:147–57.

93. Craig T, Aygören-Pürsün E, Bork K, et al. WAO guideline for the management of hereditary angioedema. World Allergy Organ J 2012;5:182–99.

Pharmacoeconomics of Orphan Disease Treatment with a Focus on Hereditary Angioedema

William R. Lumry, MD[a,b],*

KEYWORDS

- Pharmacoeconomics • Orphan disease • Hereditary angioedema • Burden
- Treatment

KEY POINTS

- Orphan diseases affect 1 in 10 individuals.
- Legislation has been successful in encouraging development of orphan disease therapies but barriers to their availability exist.
- Expenditures on orphan drugs are less than 10% of pharmaceutical expenditures and 1% of total health care costs.
- Patients with hereditary angioedema have benefited greatly from approval of novel disease-specific therapies.
- Availability of and access to these new therapies is a challenge for patients, families, and health care providers.

OVERVIEW

Hereditary angioedema (HAE) is a rare autosomal dominantly transmitted genetic disease.[1,2] It occurs in approximately 1 out of 30,000 to 80,000 individuals and affects fewer than 8000 individuals in the United States, 15,000 in North America, and 200,000 worldwide.[3,4] Although available in other countries since 1979,[5] disease-specific therapy for HAE only recently became available in the United States and North America. With the US Food and Drug Administration (FDA) approval of a human

Disclosure Statement: Dr W.R. Lumry has received clinical research grants from and serves as a consultant and advisor to BioCryst, CSL Behring, Pharming, and Shire. He provides educational programs for Pharming, CSL Behring, and Shire. He is a member of the Medical Advisory Board for the US Hereditary Angioedema Association.

[a] Internal Medicine/Allergy/Immunology Division, University of Texas Southwestern Medical School, Dallas, TX, USA; [b] AARA Research Associates, Private Practice, 10100 North Central Expressway, Suite 100, Dallas, TX 75231, USA
* Corresponding author. 10100 North Central Expressway, Suite 100, Dallas, TX 75231.
E-mail address: lumrymd@allergyspecialists.us

nanofiltered plasma-derived C1 inhibitor (C1INH) concentrate for routine prophylaxis of HAE attacks on October 10, 2008, a new era in therapy for HAE began.[6] Since 2008, 4 therapies to treat HAE attacks have received FDA approval, including a pasteurized human plasma–derived C1INH and ecallantide in 2009, icatibant in 2011, and a recombinant C1INH in 2014. These therapies are currently registered in many countries around the world (**Table 1**). (See Meng Chen and Marc Riedl's article, "Emerging Therapies in Hereditary Angioedema", in this issue.)

This burst of development and approvals has greatly benefited individuals with HAE, their families, caregivers, physicians, and health care providers.[12,13] The burden of HAE has been reduced; quality of life improved; and utilization of urgent care, emergency facilities, and hospitals decreased significantly.[14,15] Concerns have been raised, however, by health care payers in the United States and health care systems in other countries about the financial impact of these newly approved therapies on health care payment systems.[16–19] These concerns have led to barriers to and limitation of access to these potentially life-changing and lifesaving therapies.[16,17,20]

This article discusses the prevalence of orphan diseases, legislative incentives to encourage development of orphan disease therapies, and the impact of orphan disease treatment on health care payment systems. More specifically, the cost burden of HAE on patients, health care systems, and society is reviewed. The impact of availability of and access to novel and specific therapies on morbidity, mortality, and the overall burden of disease is explored. Changes in the treatment paradigms to improve effectiveness and reduce cost of treatment are presented.

ORPHAN DRUG DEVELOPMENT POLICIES AND REIMBURSEMENT ISSUES

Orphan drug policies have been established in the United States, the European Union (EU), and Japan to encourage the development of safe and effective therapies for rare diseases. The US Orphan Drug Act was enacted in 1983.[21] Under this act, a drug is given orphan designation if the disease it treats affects fewer than 200,000 individuals or if there is no reasonable expectation of profitability for the drug. Some of the incentives provided include tax credits for research costs, grants to aid in clinical research, and a 7-year marketing exclusivity for approved orphan drugs.

In 1999, the EU enacted its orphan drug policy that defines an orphan disease as a disease with 5 patients per 100,000 individuals. Research incentives are available within the EU and its member states and fees are waived for approval of the marketing application. Approved orphan drugs in the EU are given a 10-year marketing exclusivity.[22]

These policies have been successful in incentivizing companies to research and develop therapies for a wide variety of rare conditions. Before the passage of the orphan drug policies, orphan disease therapies were often neglected by pharmaceutical companies. In January, 1983, there were 38 drugs approved in the United States for orphan disorders.[23] In December 2016, 588 approved drugs are listed in the Orphan Disease Therapeutic Registry[24] and 86 designated orphan drugs approved for marketing in the EU.[25]

PREVALENCE OF ORPHAN DISEASES

There are 25 to 30 million individuals, 8% to 10% of the population of the United States, affected by 1 of the 7000 diseases designated as orphan diseases who may benefit from provisions of the Orphan Drug Act.[16,23] Treatments for these rare diseases have provided great benefits to affected individuals and their families. The high cost of many of these therapies has led to the perception by payers and society in general that treatment of orphan diseases places an inordinate burden on the health care payment systems.[16,17] This concern about excess costs of this treatment has resulted in barriers being put in place to limit access. Some of these barriers include formulary approval, high coinsurance and copayment rates, prior authorization and multiple reauthorizations, step therapy, and limits on supply and resupply of medication.[16,17,20]

Drug research and development are time-consuming and expensive propositions. The total average cost of developing and winning market approval for a new prescription drug was recently estimated to be $2.6 billion, with $1.4 billion of this amount spent on research and development.[26,27] Orphan drugs are no exception. With many fewer patients to treat, the cost to recover research and development expenditures may be high per patient treated. In 2014, the average (median) drug costs per patient per year in the United States for treatment of conditions that were not orphan was $23,331($4775) compared with $111,820 ($66,057) per the patient treated for an orphan disease.[23]

Although the cost per patient to treat an orphan disease is often high, the perception that cost of treatment of rare diseases as a whole has an inordinate impact on total pharmaceutical expenditures and health care costs is inaccurate. Analyses in the United States and the EU have shown this impact is minimal and in line with the 8% to 10% prevalence of these diseases in the population. In 2014, total expenditures for pharmaceuticals in the United States accounted for 9.8% of total health care costs of $3.0 trillion. Expenditures on orphan drugs for orphan indications was approximately $33.5 billion, representing less than 10% of pharmaceutical expenditures and 1% of the total health care expenditures.[23,28]

Despite this discrepancy between the number of drugs approved in the US and the EU, the percentage of pharmaceutical expenditures for orphan drugs in the EU was similar to the United States. Orphan drug expenditures in 17 European countries in 2011 were 3.3% of total pharmaceutical expenditures.[29] More specifically, spending was 2.5% in Sweden and 3.1% in France in 2012,[30] and 4.2% in the Netherlands in 2014.[31]

Orphan drug expenditures have been increasing over the last decade. In part, this is due to the increasing number of therapies registered and approved. In 2007, $13.3 billion was spent in the United States, accounting for 4.3% of $311 billon total expenditures for pharmaceuticals that year. By 2013, this increased to $25.8 billion, 7.7% of $337 billion spent. IMS Health's market prognosis has forecasted US total drug expenditures of $465.0 billion in 2018, with orphan drugs accounting for $44.10 billion; 9.5% of this amount represents an increase of 0.7% over 4 years.[28,32]

IMPACT OF NEW THERAPIES FOR HEREDITARY ANGIOEDEMA

Patients with HAE have benefited from approval of novel, disease-specific drugs that treat and prevent swelling attacks. The benefits include improvement in health and quality of life, increased ability to work and pursue educational and career goals, reduced disability, reduction of costly urgent care visits and hospitalizations, and longer survival.[12–14,33] The development of these drugs was made economically feasible by the orphan drug policies in the United States and the EU.

The cost of these therapies is high. In 2012, the cost of nanofiltered C1INH, Cinryze (Shire, Lexington, MA, USA) indicated for routine prophylaxis of HAE attacks when used at approved dosage and interval was $487,000 per patient, the most expensive drug for any orphan disease treated in the United States.[34] In 2015, sales of Cinryze generated the second highest revenue to a pharmaceutical company, $210,000 per patient treated, of all orphan drugs in the United States.[23] Current average wholesale

Table 1
Availability of specific treatments for hereditary angioedema across the world in 2017

Drug	Registration	Acute Treatment	Indication			Age Groups		Route
			Prophylaxis		Home-Therapy	Children	Adolescence	
			STP	LTP		<12 y	12–18 y	
pdC1NH (Berinert)[7]	EU	✓	✓	—	✓	✓	✓	IV
	US	✓	—	—	✓	✓	✓	IV
	Latin America (Brazil, Argentina, Mexico, Colombia, Chile, Puerto Rico)	✓	✓	—	✓	—	—	IV
	Australia, Canada	✓	✓	—	✓	✓	✓	IV
	Israel	✓	✓	—	✓	—	✓	IV
	Japan	✓	✓	—	✓	—	✓	IV
	South Korea	✓	✓	—	✓	✓	✓	IV
rhC1INH (Ruconest)[8]	EU	✓	—	—	✓	—	—	IV
	US	✓	—	—	✓	—	✓	IV
pdC1INH (Cinryze)[9]	EU	✓	✓	✓	✓	—	✓	IV
	US	—	—	✓	✓	—	✓	IV
	Australia, Canada, Israel	✓	✓	✓	✓	—	—	IV
Icatibant (Firazyr)[10]	EU	✓	—	—	✓	—	—	SC
	US	✓	—	—	✓	—	—	SC
	Latin America (Brazil, Argentina, Mexico, Colombia)	✓	—	—	✓	—	—	SC
	Australia, Canada	✓	—	—	✓	—	—	SC
	Israel, Kuwait, South Africa	✓	—	—	✓	—	—	SC
Ecallantide (Kalbitor)[11]	EU	—	—	—	—	—	—	SC
	US	✓	—	—	—	—	✓	SC
Attenuated Androgens	EU	—	✓	✓	✓	—	✓	Oral
	US	—	—	✓	✓	—	—	Oral
	Latin America (Brazil, Argentina, Mexico, Colombia)	✓	—	✓	✓	—	—	Oral

Drug	Region							Route
Transexamic Acid	EU	✓	✓			✓		Oral
	US							Oral
	Latin America (Brazil, Argentina, Mexico, Colombia)	✓		✓				Oral
Epsilon Amino Caproic Acid	EU							Oral
	US							Oral
	Latin America (Brazil, Argentina, Mexico, Colombia)							Oral
Icatibant (Firazyr)[10]	EU	✓ ✓ ✓		✓ ✓ ✓				SC
	US	✓ ✓		✓ ✓				SC
	Latin America (Brazil, Argentina, Mexico, Colombia)	✓ ✓ ✓ ✓ ✓		✓ ✓ ✓ ✓ ✓				SC
	Australia							SC
	Canada							SC
	Israel							SC
	Kuwait							SC
	South Africa							SC
Ecallantide (Kalbitor)[11]	EU	✓				✓	✓	SC
	US							IV
	Latin America (Brazil, Argentina, Mexico, Colombia)							
Attenuated Androgens	EU	✓	✓ ✓	✓ ✓ ✓		✓		Oral
	US		✓ ✓	✓ ✓				Oral
	Latin America (Brazil, Argentina, Mexico, Colombia)	✓		✓				Oral
Transexamic Acid	EU	✓	✓			✓	✓	Oral
	US							Oral
	Latin America (Brazil, Argentina, Mexico, Colombia)	✓		✓				Oral
Epsilon Amino Caproic Acid	EU					✓	✓	Oral
	US							Oral
	Latin America (Brazil, Argentina, Mexico, Colombia)							Oral

Abbreviations: IV, intravenous; LTP, Long term (routine) prophylaxis; SC, subcutaneous; STP, Short term prophylaxis.

prices for treatments of acute attacks range from $5000 to more than $10,000 per attack treated. The cost of these therapies is generally lower outside of the United States, with some national health systems able to acquire them at a significant discount to United States prices.

The cost of not adequately treating HAE is also high. These costs include not only the direct cost of providing medical care to these patients but also the indirect cost of the disease on patients, their family, and on society. Patients with HAE consume more health care and are more costly to the health care system, even if the costs of the newer medications are not included. In a United Kingdom (UK) study, the cost of care for a patient was 160% for primary care and 447% for secondary care, even if the costs of specialist care and medications were excluded.[35] Patients with HAE and their caregivers miss a significant amount of time from work and school, are often less productive at work, and may be unable to achieve their educational and career goals, or even maintain employment, as a result of their attacks.[33,36]

COST OF HEREDITARY ANGIOEDEMA CARE BEFORE 2008 IN THE UNITED STATES

Disease-specific therapies for HAE were not available in the United States before 2008. This provides an opportunity to review costs and impact of the disease before current therapies became available. An Internet survey completed by members of the US Hereditary Angioedema Association (HAEA) in 2007 found that patients experienced an average of 26.9 swelling attacks per year, lasting 61.3 hours each. More than 80% were considered moderate to severe in intensity.[36] Total annual cost of having and treating HAE was also assessed in this survey.[37] The average annual cost per patient was $44,597. Cost varied depending on the severity of the disease, ranging from $11,587 for mildly affected patients to $28,764 and $104,857, respectively, for those moderately or severely affected. The total mean annual expenditure per HAE patient of $44,597 included direct medical costs of $29,177, which comprised $17,381 for hospital admissions, $2827 for emergency department (ED) visits, $3777 for outpatient care, and $5194 for medications; and indirect costs of $15,420, including $5157 for reduced productivity, $6417 for reduced income, $3402 for missed work, and $4444 for travel and childcare.[37] Accounting for inflation, the average annual cost per patient in 2016 dollars would be $62,440.

ED usage and hospitalization before 2008 was high because only supportive treatment was available, including intravenous fluids, antiemetics, analgesics, and airway support. In 2007, there were 2705 ED visits with HAE as the primary diagnosis, with 40.9% resulting in hospitalization. At a mean cost of $1479 per ED visit, $3,727,080 was spent in the United States for urgent care.[38] Between 2004 and 2007, there were 10,125 hospitalizations in which HAE was the primary or secondary diagnosis. The average length of stay was 5.1 days and the average cost per hospitalization was $8383, resulting in $21,220,000 annual expenditure for hospital services.[39]

BURDEN OF DISEASE

In addition to the direct cost of care, indirect costs must be considered. Missed time from work or school, decreased productivity at work, and loss of opportunity are significant costs to the patient and society. Patients report a decrease of productivity at the job due to HAE.[37] A national audit in the UK of patients with HAE and acquired angioedema revealed that patients lost on average 9 days of work per year, ranging from 0 to 43 days.[40] An EU study of the socioeconomic burden of HAE revealed both patients and caregivers were affected, with each losing an average of 20 days from work or school per year.[33,41]

Loss of educational and career opportunity is commonly reported. In the HAEA survey conducted in 2007, 57% of HAE patients reported having career advancement hindered, 69% thought that they could not consider certain types of jobs because of their disease, 100% thought that educational advancement had been hindered, 55% had to limit their educational choices, and 48% had not achieved the level of education that they desired.[36] Even after disease-specific therapies became available, decreased opportunity is still a problem. In the EU socioeconomic burden of disease report published in 2014 after current therapies became available, 42% patients reported their educational advancement was hindered, 40% were prevented from applying for certain jobs, 36% thought that their career advancement was diminished, 9% switched positions within their company, and 10% left their position permanently because of this disabling disease.[33] HAE patients also suffer from anxiety and depression at much higher rates than the normal population. Results from 2 independent studies suggest that between 14% and 43% of patients of HAE experience clinically significant depression, further adding to their disability.[36,42]

A fatal HAE attack with loss of an individual from both the work force and society is the ultimate burden of this disease, and results in significant hardship both socially and economically to the patient's family and society. Unfortunately, patients with HAE continue to succumb to this treatable disease. In a review of all US death certificates from 1999 to 2010, HAE was considered a contributing factor or the underlying cause of death in 600 people, with 270 of these deaths directly attributed to HAE.[43] In a German study that included 728 subjects from 182 families with HAE type I and type II, 214 deaths were recorded. The mean age of death from an HAE attack was 40.6 years.[44]

INNOVATIVE TREATMENT PARADIGMS

Although disease-specific treatments for HAE are expensive, appropriate and timely treatment decreases ED visits, hospitalizations, lost time from school and work, and prevents death, lowering the overall cost of the disease to the health care system and to society. ED visits and hospitalization for supportive treatment were the norm before availability of home and self-administration of treatment.[36] Self-administration of treatment and prevention of attacks is safe, effective, and encouraged. Patients can accurately recognize and safely self-treat HAE attacks, leading to earlier treatment, earlier resolution of symptoms, decreased ED and hospital visits, improved quality of life, and cost savings.[15,41,45–49]

Innovative treatment paradigms may further lower the cost and the burden of disease. Italian HAE subjects who self-administered C1INH concentrate decreased their mean annual number of hospitalizations from 16.8 to 2.1, time to administration of treatment from 3.2 to 1.9 hours, time to symptom improvement from 84 to 54 minutes, time to symptom resolution from 12.8 to 10.8 hours, and number of missed days of work or school from 23.3 to 7.1 compared with therapy administered in a hospital or ED. The total cost of therapy, including direct and indirect cost, was approximately 30,010 Euros ($40,500) per subjects when the therapy was administered in a hospital or clinic setting, and 26,621 Euros ($36,000) when treatment was administered at home. This represented a savings of 11% or 57,619 Euros ($78,000) for the 17 subjects reported in the study.[50]

Spanish investigators estimated patients who self-treated their HAE attacks with icatibant compared with health care setting administration would save an average of 121 Euros ($170) per attack in direct and indirect costs, a 9.2% decrease in costs. Reduction in direct costs accounted for 74% of the savings. This would achieve an annual health system savings of 551,371 Euros ($772,000).[51] A US study reported a

$650,000 savings when 249 HAE attacks over 5 months were treated with ecallantide given at home by an infusion nurse compared with the cost of treating these attacks in the ED or hospital.[52] In the UK, home administration of icatibant compared with hospital administration of C1INH saved $861 to $1167 per attack.[53]

In Demark, 80 HAE subjects were followed prospectively for 10 years. By 2012, 49% were self-administering C1NH or icatibant, with 84% reduction in ED visits. In the self-treated subjects, there was no need for tracheotomy, no deaths reported, and an improved quality of life in all physical and psychological domains. Despite a 300% increase in use of newer so-called high-cost treatments, the cost to treat an average of 36 attacks per subject per year was manageable at $16,766.[49]

Unfortunately, in many countries, implementation of a home or self-administration policy is not possible. In Japan, Greece, and most of Eastern Europe, acute therapies are only available at the hospital or specialty clinics, if available at all. In Brazil and Mexico, home therapy is available but is not reimbursed (personal communication).

Specific treatments for HAE attacks are available in many countries (see **Table 1**). Treatments to prevent attacks are less widely available. What is not obvious from this **Table 1** is that, although these treatments may be registered and approved for marketing in a particular country, they may not be accessible to the patients that need them. Barriers to access include requirement for health care system or judicial approval, availability only in specialized treatment centers or hospitals, limits on reimbursement, and limits on number of treatments allowed or resupply of medication to providers or patients.

An example of this problem is found in Argentina. Members of the Argentine Hereditary Angioedema Patient Association completed questionnaires about the availability and their access to HAE treatments in 2009, 2013, and 2016. Despite C1INH being registered and approved for treatment of HAE attacks before 2009, C1INH was available to only 26% of those responding to the survey in 2009. This increased to 55% by 2016. Only 10% had access to icatibant in 2016. Reimbursement for these medications in 2016 was also a challenge, with only 64% reimbursed at 100% and 19% having no reimbursement available at all. Most patients received treatment from health personnel or at the hospital and more than 50% reported not receiving treatment until their attack was severely painful. Reordering and resupply of medication was difficult for 66% of patients, with only 20% reporting a fast replacement and 53% able to obtain replacement within 10 days.[54]

Despite the advances in the treatment of HAE, with availability of new, effective, on-demand, and prophylactic treatments, many of these medications are not approved in many countries around the world. Even if approved, they are not accessible by the patients who need them. Despite improvement of treatment outcomes and cost savings when the treatment is self-administered or given in the home setting, on-demand therapies are only accessible in hospital and clinic settings in many countries.

SUMMARY

Orphan drug policies are in place to encourage development of safe and effective therapies for orphan diseases. With a limited number of patients to treat, the cost per patient of orphan drugs to recover research and development costs is high. Orphan diseases affect approximately 8% to 10% of the population. Overall, expenditures for drugs to treat orphan diseases remain proportionately less than the incidence of these diseases in the population. Expenditures for orphan drugs are currently less than 10% of pharmaceutical expenditures and 1% of the total health care costs in the United States. Despite these facts, payers in the United States and health care authorities around the world perceive that care for orphan diseases places an inordinate burden on their payment systems and have put barriers in place to limit their use.

Orphan drugs benefit many people with previously underserved orphan diseases. These drugs offer significant value to patients and society in terms of improvements in health; reduced disability; increased productivity, including the ability to continue working; reduced health care utilization; improved quality of life; and survival. Patients with HAE are not an exception and have benefited greatly. Availability of new and novel therapies to treat and prevent swelling attacks have dramatically decreased the burden of disease in this heretofore underserved population. Prudent therapeutic choices, utilization of new treatment paradigms, and improvement in availability and accessibility of these new therapies will continue to improve the lives of patients with HAE. Continued coverage of these life-altering and lifesaving therapies should continue and barriers to access should be addressed.

The conversation about the high cost for the benefit obtained of orphan drugs with payers, society, and patients needs to change to recognition of the benefits of timely and appropriate care. Clinicians need to solve the access problem by working with health systems, patients, and their advocates on the most cost-effective and efficient ways to deliver this care. Clinicians must continue to disseminate knowledge regarding benefits to patients and to society of effective and safe treatments for HAE and all rare diseases.

REFERENCES

1. Agostoni A, Cicardi M. Hereditary and acquired C1-inhibitor deficiency: biological and clinical characteristics in 235 patients. Medicine 1992;71:206–15.
2. Frank MM, Gelfand JA, Atkinson JP. Hereditary angioedema: the clinical syndrome and its management. Ann Intern Med 1976;84:580–93.
3. Zuraw BL. Clinical practice: hereditary angioedema. N Engl J Med 2008;359: 1027–36 [Review] [53 refs].
4. Cicardi M, Agostoni A. Hereditary angioedema. N Engl J Med 1996;334:1666–7.
5. Bowen T, Cicardi M, Farkas H, et al. 2010 International consensus algorithm for the diagnosis, therapy and management of hereditary angioedema. Allergy Asthma Clin Immunol 2010;6(1):24.
6. Lunn M, Santos C, Craig T. Cinryze™ as the first approved C1 inhibitor in the USA for the treatment of hereditary angioedema: approval, efficacy and safety. J Blood Med 2010;1:163–70.
7. Berinert prescribing information. CSL Behring. Available at: http://labeling. cslbehring.com/PI/US/Berinert/EN/Berinert-Prescribing-Information.pdf. Accessed December 2016.
8. Ruconest prescribing information. Pharming pharmaceuticals. Available at: https:// shared.salix.com/shared/pi/ruconest-pi.pdf. Accessed December 01, 2016.
9. Cinryze prescribing information. Shire. Available at: http://pi.shirecontent.com/PI/ PDFs/Cinryze_USA_ENG.pdf. Accessed December 2016.
10. Firazyr prescribing information. Shire. Available at: http://labeling.cslbehring.com/ PI/US/Berinert/EN/Berinert-Prescribing-Information.pdf. Accessed December 01, 2016.
11. Kalbitor prescribing information. Dyax Corporation. Available at: http://www.kalbitor. com/hcp/rems/pdf/KalbitorFullPrescribingInformation.pdf. Accessed December 01, 2016.

12. Christiansen SC, Bygum A, Banerji A, et al. Before and after, the impact of available on-demand treatment for HAE. Allergy Asthma Proc 2015;36(2):145–50.
13. Longhurst H, Bygum A. The Humanistic, Societal, and Pharmaco-economic Burden of Angioedema. Clin Rev Allergy Immunol 2016;51(2):230–9.
14. Banerji A, Busse P, Christiansen SC, et al. Current state of hereditary angioedema management: a patient survey. Allergy Asthma Proc 2015;36(3):213–7.
15. Longhurst HJ, Farkas H, Craig T, et al. HAE international home therapy consensus document. Allergy Asthma Clin Immunol 2010;6:22.
16. Handfield R, Feldstein J. Insurance companies' perspectives on the orphan drug pipeline. Am Health Drug Benefits 2013;6(9):589–98.
17. Hyde R, Dobrovolny D. Orphan drug pricing and payer management in the United States: are we approaching the tipping point? Am Health Drug Benefits 2010;3(1):15–23.
18. Cardarelli W. Managed care implications of hereditary angioedema. Am J Manag Care 2013;19(7 Suppl):s119–24.
19. Morrow T. Insurers will find icatibant lifesaving but expensive treatment. Managed care once again faces the all-too-familiar debate about cost and benefit. Manag Care 2011;20(11):63–4.
20. Robinson SW, Brantley K, Liow C, et al. An early examination of access to select orphan drugs treating rare diseases in health insurance exchange plans. J Manag Care Spec Pharm 2014;20(10):997–1004.
21. Food and drug administration. Orphan drug act. Silver Spring (MD) FDA. Available at: http://www.fda.gov/RegulatoryInformation/Legislation/Significant AmendmentstotheFDCAct/OrphanDrugAct/. Accessed December 01, 2016.
22. Regulation (EC) No 141/2000 of the European parliament and of the council of 16 December 1999 on orphan medicinal products official journal L 018, 22/01/2000 P. 0001 – 0005. Available at: http://eur-lex.europa.eu/legal-content/EN/TXT/?uri=uriserv:OJ.L_.2000.018.01.0001.01.ENG&toc=OJ:L:2000:018:TOC. Accessed December 01, 2016.
23. EvaluatePharma orphan drug report 2015. 3rd Edition.2015. Available at: http://info. evaluategroup.com/rs/607-YGS-364/images/EPOD15.pdf. Accessed December 1, 2016.
24. Food and drug administration. Orphan drug approval list. Silver Spring (MD): FDA. Available at: http://www.accessdata.fda.gov/scripts/opdlisting/oopd/list Result.cfm. Accessed December 01, 2016.
25. Orphanet: list of orphan drugs in Europe. Available at: http://www.orpha.net/orphacom/ cahiers/docs/GB/list_of_orphan_drugs_in_europe.pdf. Accessed December 01, 2016.
26. DiMasi JA, Grabowski HG, Hansen RW. Innovation in the pharmaceutical industry: new estimates of R&D costs. Boston: Tufts Center for the Study of Drug Development; 2014. Available at: http://csdd.tufts.edu/news/complete_ story/cost_study_press_event_webcast.
27. Avorn J. The $2.6 billion pill – methodologic and policy considerations. N Engl J Med 2015;372:1877–9.
28. Divino V, Dekoven M, Kleinrock M, et al. Orphan drug expenditures in the United States: a historical and prospective analysis, 2007-18. Health Aff 2016;35(9): 1588–94.
29. Schey C, Milanova T, Hutchings A. Estimating the budget impact of orphan medicines in Europe: 2010–2020. Orphanet J Rare Dis 2011;6:62.
30. Hutchings A, Schey C, Dutton R, et al. Estimating the budget impact of orphan drugs in Sweden and France 2013–2020. Orphanet J Rare Dis 2014;9:22.

31. Kanters TA, Steenhoek A, Hakkaart L. Orphan drugs expenditure in the Netherlands in the period 2006–2012. Orphanet J Rare Dis 2014;9:154.
32. IMS Health. Market prognosis 2014– 2018, USA. London: IMS Health; 2014.
33. Aygören-Pürsün E, Bygum A, Beusterien K, et al. Socioeconomic burden of hereditary angioedema: results from the hereditary angioedema burden of illness study in Europe. Orphanet J Rare Dis 2014;9:99–108.
34. Tilles SA, Borish L, Cohen JP. Management of hereditary angioedema in 2012: scientific and pharmacoeconomic perspectives. Ann Allergy Asthma Immunol 2013;110(2):70–4.
35. Helbert M, Holbrook T, Drogon E, et al. Exploring cost and burden of illness of HAE in the UK. Liverpool (England): Poster UKPIN; 2013.
36. Lumry WR, Castaldo AJ, Vernon MK, et al. The humanistic burden of hereditary angioedema: impact on health-related quality of life, productivity, and depression. Allergy Asthma Proc 2010;31(5):407–14.
37. Wilson DA, Bork K, Shea EP, et al. Economic costs associated with acute attacks and long-term management of hereditary angioedema. Ann Allergy Asthma Immunol 2010;104(4):314–20.
38. Zilberberg MD, Nathanson BH, Jacobsen T, et al. Descriptive epidemiology of hereditary angioedema emergency department visits in the United States, 2006-2007. Allergy Asthma Proc 2011;32(5):390–4.
39. Zilberberg MD, Nathanson BH, Jacobsen T, et al. Descriptive epidemiology of hereditary angioedema hospitalizations in the United States, 2004–2007. Allergy Asthma Proc 2011;32(3):248–54.
40. Jolles S, Williams P, Carne E, et al. A UK national audit of hereditary and acquired angioedema. Clin Exp Immunol 2014;175(1):59–67.
41. Hernández Fernandez de Rojas D, Ibañez E, Longhurst H, et al, IOS Study Group. Treatment of HAE attacks in the icatibant outcome survey: an analysis of icatibant self-administration versus administration by health care professionals. Int Arch Allergy Immunol 2015;167:21–8.
42. Fouche AS, Saunders EF, Craig T. Depression and anxiety in patients with hereditary angioedema. Ann Allergy Asthma Immunol 2014;112(4):371–5.
43. Kim SJ, Brooks JC, Sheikh J, et al. Angioedema deaths in the United States, 1979-2010. Ann Allergy Asthma Immunol 2014;113(6):630–4.
44. Bork K, Hardt J, Witzke G. Fatal laryngeal attacks and mortality in hereditary angioedema due to C1-INH deficiency. J Allergy Clin Immunol 2012;130(3):692–7.
45. Aberer W, Maurer M, Reshef A, et al. Open-label, multicenter study of self-administered icatibant for attacks of hereditary angioedema. Allergy 2014;69: 305–14.
46. Tourangeau LM, Castaldo AJ, Davis DK, et al. Safety and efficacy of physician-supervised self-managed C1 inhibitor replacement therapy. Int Arch Allergy Immunol 2012;157:417–24.
47. Maurer M, Aberer W, Bouillet L, et al. Hereditary angioedema attacks resolve faster and are shorter after early icatibant treatment. PLoS One 2013;8:e53773.
48. Levi M, Choi G, Picavet C, et al. Self-administration of C1-inhibitor concentrate in patients with hereditary or acquired angioedema caused by C1-inhibitor deficiency. J Allergy Clin Immunol 2006;117(4):904–8.
49. Bygum A. Hereditary angioedema - consequences of a new treatment paradigm in Denmark. Acta Derm Venereol 2014;94(4):436–41.
50. Petraroli A, Squeglia V, Di Paola N, et al. Home therapy with plasma-derived c1 inhibitor: a strategy to improve clinical outcomes and costs in hereditary angioedema. Int Arch Allergy Immunol 2015;166(4):259–66.

51. Blasco AJ, Lázaro P, Caballero T, et al. Social costs of icatibant self-administration vs. health professional-administration in the treatment of hereditary angioedema in Spain. Health Econ Rev 2013;3(1):2.
52. Speciality pharmacy news. 2012; 9(7): 9–11.
53. NHS commissioning board clinical commissioning policy: treatment of acute attacks in hereditary angioedema. Available at: https://www.england.nhs.uk/wp-content/uploads/2013/04/b09-p-b.pdf. Accessed December 01, 2016.
54. Menendez A, Malbran A. C1inh-Hae. A web based poll on accessibility to acute attack treatments in Argentina. Poster presented at Third HAEI Global Conference. Madrid, Spain, May 19–22, 2016.

Moving?

Make sure your subscription moves with you!

To notify us of your new address, find your **Clinics Account Number** (located on your mailing label above your name), and contact customer service at:

Email: journalscustomerservice-usa@elsevier.com

800-654-2452 (subscribers in the U.S. & Canada)
314-447-8871 (subscribers outside of the U.S. & Canada)

Fax number: 314-447-8029

Elsevier Health Sciences Division
Subscription Customer Service
3251 Riverport Lane
Maryland Heights, MO 63043

*To ensure uninterrupted delivery of your subscription, please notify us at least 4 weeks in advance of move.

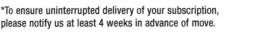

Printed and bound by CPI Group (UK) Ltd, Croydon, CR0 4YY

07/10/2024

01040502-0018